More

More Chicken Soup

& · OTHER · FOLK · REMEDIES ·

REVISED EDITION

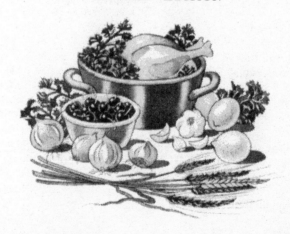

JOAN WILEN AND LYDIA WILEN

ILLUSTRATIONS BY
ELIZABETH KODA-CALLAN

Ballantine Books • New York

The information contained in this book is based upon the research and experiences of the authors and the many contributors who shared their experiences and expertise. It is not intended as a substitute for consulting with your health-care provider.

The publisher and authors are not responsible for any consequences resulting from the use of any of the suggestions or preparations discussed in this book. All matters pertaining to your physical health should be supervised by your health-care professional.

Seeking more than one or two opinions is not a sign of insecurity, but a sign of wisdom.

A Ballantine Book
The Random House Publishing Group

Published in the United States by Ballantine Books, an imprint of The Random House Publishing Group, a division of Random House, Inc., New York, and simultaneously in Canada by Random House of Canada Limited, Toronto. Originally published in slightly different form by The Random House Publishing Group, a division of Random House, Inc., in 1984.

Ballantine and colophon are registered trademarks of Random House, Inc.

www.ballantinebooks.com

ISBN: 978-0-345-44061-7

Cover design by Min Choi
Cover illustration by Gamboa Publishing

Manufactured in the United States of America

Revised Edition: September 2000

10 9 8 7 6 5 4 3 2

MORE CHICKEN SOUP & OTHER FOLK REMEDIES

*is dedicated to people who are
dedicated to helping heal others.*

Contents

x · Contents

Acknowledgments

SPECIAL THANKS to family and friends who have offered us their loving support, good wishes, and remedies.

J. Walter Allen
Larry Ashmead
Tisi Aylward
Nancy Barrett
Tom Bergeron
Cynthia Bernabach
Jane Biberman
Bill Mason Bivens
Heather Brodhead
Ted Brown
Father Sam Bungo
Patricia Burke
Myles P. Burton
Barbara Carpenter
Jonathan Feldman
Alyce Finell
Ronald E. Franzmeier
Gotham Group of Hadassah
Linda Guss
Anne Hardy
Candace Harmon
Angela Harris and Family
Don Hauptman
Maddie Henri
Erika Holzer
Hank Holzer
Karen Horbatt
Eric Stephen Jacobs

Hillary Jacobs
Laurie Jacoby
Arlen Hollis Kane
Avril LaCour
Ruth Landa
Ruth Lesser
Jena Levinson
Lee Levinson
Nick Malekos
Beverly Marcus
Blanche Miller
Dr. Marie Neag
Martha Neag
John Nicholas
George Nider
Eileen Nock
B.L. Ochman & Sam
Robert Pardi
Richard A. Perozzi
Janine Pietrucha
Otto Pietrucha
Andy Port
Chipp Prosnit
Diane Rappoport
Larry Royce
Michael L. Samuels
Mae Schenk and Family
Barbara Schulick

Paul Schulick
Dorothy Senerchia
Rudy Shur
Owen Spann
Dick Syatt
Helen Tierney

Allen Tobias
John Turner
Judy Twersky
Robert Weinstein
Linda Wilen
Teena Wrobel

BIG THANKS to all of the television shows, radio shows, newspapers, magazines, and Websites that have and continue to help us get the word out about us, our work, and our books.

Our gratitude to Leona Nevler for helping us start it all with our first folk remedy book. Our heartfelt appreciation to all of the people who bought copies of that first book, making this sequel possible.

Special thanks to Joelle Delbourgo for being the driving force behind the original MORE CHICKEN SOUP, and to our (then) editor, Michelle Russell.

The driving force behind this new-millennium version is our present editor, Elizabeth Zack. We love that she loves to edit, and we thank her for her patience, input, and passion.

Many of the NOTES, CAUTIONS, and WARNINGS throughout this book are a reflection of the fastidious scrutiny of Ray C. Wunderlich, Jr., M.D., who reviewed every remedy with your well-being in mind. Dr. Wunderlich has been exceptionally generous with his time, knowledge, and even some of his own remedies that he graciously shared. We feel blessed to know this healer, teacher, and the only other person in our time zone whom we won't awaken if we call at two A.M.

Introduction

When we were growing up in Brooklyn, each winter my mom would crochet little drawstring bags and my dad would see to it they were filled with camphor, which he then insisted we wear around our necks. Daddy was sure that it would prevent us from catching colds. We reeked so from the camphor, none of our friends would come near us, and we didn't catch their colds. Daddy was right.

When we'd walk into a room, the camphor smell was so strong that we'd joke, "We weren't born, we were just taken out of storage."

That camphor was our introduction to folk remedies . . . along with honey and lemon for a sore throat, sugar water for the hiccups, horseradish to clear the sinuses, garlic for a whole bunch of things, and chicken soup for everything else.

Our mom made the world's best chicken soup . . . when she wasn't crocheting little drawstring bags for the camphor. In fact, the soup recipe is in our first book, *Chicken Soup & Other Folk Remedies*.

In this book, we have a chicken soup recipe that's from a doctor. It's so potent . . . How potent is it? It's so potent that the dosage is only two tablespoons of it at a time. Just about all the rest of the remedies in this book require one or two ingredients; some require nothing except your concentration and an acupressure point.

When we wrote our first folk remedy book, we limited ourselves to ingredients everyone was familiar with, and probably had in their kitchen. In the original version of this, our second book, we were a little more daring. We introduced our readers to some fruits, vegetables, vitamins, minerals, and herbs that were new to them and not always easy to find. That was then. Now health food stores are in every town, supermarkets have health food sections, greengrocers are in every neighborhood, and whatever is not down your block or on your corner, you can find at your fingertips on the Internet. (Be sure to check out our "Sources" chapter.)

So now that everything is readily available, you can learn to take care of yourself, feel great, and practice preventive medicine. We've added a valuable chapter: Our "Sensational Six Superfoods." These extraordinary edibles have the power to help protect, improve, save, and extend people's lives.

To find the most beneficial and tastiest ways to eat these foods, we did a lot of research and experimenting. We soaked, scrubbed, grated, minced, diced, spiced, blended, whipped, whisked, powdered, peeled, cooked, baked, boiled, roasted, toasted, and tested, and came up with simple suggestions for incorporating these foods into your daily diet.

It was quite an education for both of us. Once, while experimenting with bee pollen, we knew that Joan had taken too much when she had this uncontrollable urge to fling herself against a screen door.

But seriously . . .

To ensure your safety, a medical doctor has reviewed every remedy in the book and, while he still may be scratching his head at the effectiveness of some of the more unconventional remedies, he concluded that they may not always help, but they certainly wouldn't hurt.

Please, for your own well-being, and for our peace of mind, be sure to consult a health professional whom you trust before starting any self-help health treatment.

Our home remedy suggestions should not take the place of professional health care that may be needed for certain ailments and for persistent symptoms.

Please know that we do not have formal medical training. We are not prescribing treatment. We're writers, reporting on what has worked for people who have shared their remedies from generation to generation, up to and including the present. We are also reporting the findings of scientific research in laboratories throughout the world.

Thank you for reading our book.

Every good wish for your good health!
The Wilen Sisters
~ Joan & Lydia ~
P.O. Box 230416
Ansonia Station
New York, NY 10023-0416

More Chicken Soup

& · OTHER · FOLK · REMEDIES ·

Preparation Guide

‡ BARLEY

Hippocrates, the father of medicine, felt that everyone should drink barley water daily to maintain good health. Barley is rich in iron and vitamin B. It is said to help prevent tooth decay and hair loss, improve fingernails and toenails, and help heal ulcers, diarrhea, and bronchial spasms.

Pearl or pearled barley has been milled. During the milling process, the double outer husk is removed, along with its nutrients. A less refined version is pot or Scotch barley. Once it's gone through a less severe milling process, part of the bran layer remains, along with some of the nutrients. Hulled barley, with only the outer, inedible hull removed, is rich in dietary fiber, and has more iron, trace minerals, and four times the thiamine (B_1) of pearled barley. It's available at some health food stores, as is Scotch barley. If you can't get either, you will be able to get pearl barley at your supermarket.

BARLEY WATER: Boil 2 ounces of barley in 6 cups of water (distilled water if possible) until there's about half the water—3 cups—left in the pot. Strain. If necessary, add honey and lemon to taste.

‡ COCONUT MILK

To get the milk in the easiest way possible, you need an ice pick or a screwdriver (Phillips, if possible), and a hammer. The coconut has three little black eyelike bald spots on it. Place the ice pick or screwdriver in the middle of one black spot, then hammer the end of it so that it pierces the coconut. Repeat the procedure with the other two black spots and then pour out the coconut milk. The hammer alone should then do the trick on the rest of the coconut. Watch your fingers! (Also watch your figure. Coconut meat is high in saturated fat.)

‡ EYEWASH

REMINDER: Always remove contact lenses before doing an eyewash.

You'll need an eye cup (available at drugstores). Carefully pour just-boiled water over the cup to clean it. Then, without contaminating the rim or inside surfaces of the cup, fill it half full with whichever eyewash you've selected. Apply the cup tightly to the eye to prevent spillage, then tilt your head backward. Open your eyelid wide and rotate your eyeball to thoroughly wash the eye. Use the same procedure with the other eye.

‡ GARLIC JUICE

When a remedy calls for garlic juice, peel a clove of garlic, mince it finely onto a piece of cheesecloth, then squeeze the juice out of it. A garlic press will make the job easier.

‡ GINGER TEA

Peel or scrub a nub of fresh ginger and cut it into 3 to 5 quarter-size pieces. Pour just-boiled water over it and let it steep for five to ten minutes. If you want strong ginger tea, *grate* a piece of ginger, then steep it, strain it, and drink it. TV personality and chef Ainsley Harriott told us that he freezes ginger, making it easier to grate.

‡ HERBAL BATH

Besides offering a good relaxing time, the herbal bath can be extremely healing. The volatile oils of the herbs are activated by the heat of the water, which also opens your pores, allowing for absorption of the herbs. As you enjoy the bath, you're inhaling the herbs (aromatherapy), which pass through the nervous system to the brain, benefiting both mind and body.

HERBAL BATH DIRECTIONS: Simply take a handful of one or a combination of dried or fresh herbs and place them in the center of a white handkerchief. Secure the herbs in the handkerchief by turning it into a little knapsack. Toss the herb-filled knapsack into the tub and let the hot water fill the tub until it reaches the level you want. When the water cools enough for you to sit comfortably, do so.

After your bath, open the handkerchief and spread the herbs out to dry. You can use them a couple times more.

Instead of using dried or fresh herbs, you can use herbal essential oils. Oils cause the tub to be slippery. Be extra careful getting out of the tub, and be sure to clean the tub thoroughly after you've taken the bath.

‡ HERBAL TEA

Place a teaspoon of the herb, or the herbal tea bag, in a glass or ceramic cup and pour just-boiled water over it. (The average water-to-herb ratio is 6 to 8 ounces of water to 1 round teaspoon of herb. There are exceptions, so be sure to read the directions on the herbal tea package.)

According to the herbal tea company Lion Cross, never use water that has been boiled before. The first boiling releases oxygen and the second boiling results in "flat," lifeless tea.

Cover the cup and let the tea steep for the amount of time suggested on the package. The general rule of thumb is: steep about three minutes for flowers and soft leaves; about five minutes for seeds and leaves; about ten minutes for hard seeds, roots, and barks. Of course, the longer the tea steeps, the stronger it gets.

Strain the tea, or remove the tea bag. If you need to sweeten it, use raw honey (never use sugar because it is said to negate the value of most herbs), and when it's cool enough, drink it slowly.

‡ ONION

The onion is in the same plant family as garlic and is almost as versatile. The ancient Egyptians looked at the onion as the symbol of the universe. It has been regarded as a universal healing food, used to treat earaches, colds, fever, wounds, diarrhea, insomnia, warts, and the list goes on. It is believed that a cut onion in a sickroom disinfects the air, as it absorbs the germs in that room. Half an onion will help absorb the smell of a just-painted room. With that in mind, you may not want to use a cut piece of onion that has been in the kitchen for more than a day, unless you wrap it in plastic wrap and refrigerate it.

ONION JUICE: When a remedy calls for onion juice, grate an onion, put the gratings in a piece of cheesecloth, and squeeze out the juice.

‡ POTATOES

Raw, peeled, boiled, grated, and mashed potatoes; potato water; and potato poultices all help heal, according to American, English, and Irish folk medicine. In fact, a popular nineteenth-century Irish saying was, "Only two things in this world are too serious to be jested on: potatoes and matrimony."

The skin or peel of the potato is richer in fiber, iron,

potassium, calcium, phosphorus, zinc, and C and B vitamins than the inside of the potato. Always leave the skin on when preparing potato water, but scrub it well.

Do not use potatoes that have a green tinge. The greenish coloring is a warning that there may be a high concentration of solanine, a toxic alkaloid that can affect nerve impulses and cause vomiting, cramps, and diarrhea. The same goes for potatoes that have started to sprout. They're a no-no.

POTATO WATER: Scrub 2 medium-size potatoes (use organic whenever possible) and cut them in half. Put the 4 halves in a pot with 4 cups of water (filtered, spring, or distilled, if possible) and bring to a boil. Lower the flame a little and let it cook for thirty minutes. Take out the potatoes (eating them is optional) and save the water. Most remedies say to drink 2 cups of potato water. Refrigerate the leftover water for next time.

‡ POULTICES

Poultices are usually made with vegetables, fruit, or herbs that are either minced, chopped, grated, crushed or mashed, and sometimes cooked. These ingredients are then wrapped in a clean fabric—cheesecloth, white cotton, unbleached muslin—and applied externally to the affected area.

A poultice is most effective when moist. When the poultice dries out, it should be changed—the cloth as well as the ingredients.

Whenever possible, use fresh fruits, vegetables, or herbs. If these are unavailable, then use dried herbs. To soften herbs, pour hot water over them. Do not let herbs steep in water that's still boiling, unless the remedy specifies to do it. Boiling most herbs will diminish their healing powers.

Let's use comfrey as an example of a typical poultice.

Cut a piece of cloth twice the size of the area it will cover. If you're using a fresh leaf, wash it with cool water, then crush it in your hand. Place the leaf on one half of the cloth and fold over the other half. If you are making a poultice with dried comfrey root and leaves, pour hot water over the herb, then place the softened herb down the length of the cloth, about two inches from the edge. Roll the cloth around the herb so that it won't spill out and place it on the affected body part. Gently wrap an Ace bandage or another piece of cloth around the poultice to hold it in place and to keep in the moisture.

‡ SAUERKRAUT

Sauerkraut is fermented cabbage that has been a popular folk medicine throughout the world for centuries. The lactic acid in sauerkraut is said to encourage the growth of friendly bacteria and help destroy enemy bacteria in the large intestine (where many people believe disease may begin) and in other parts of the digestive tract. Sauerkraut is rich in vitamin B_6—which is important for brain and nervous system functions—and high in calcium—for healthy teeth and bones. In fact, in the hills of western Germany, it is reported that sauerkraut is used as a snack for children, to help prevent tooth decay and heal bad skin conditions.

The sauerkraut that comes in cans has been processed, and this may destroy its valuable properties. It is for that reason you should eat sauerkraut cold from the refrigerator, at room temperature, or after it's been warmed over a very low flame. Overheating may destroy the lactic acid and beneficial enzymes.

You can buy raw sauerkraut in jars in health food stores, or out of barrels in some ethnic stores. You can also make your own sauerkraut.

Ingredients and Supplies:
1 large head of white cabbage (about 8 cups when shredded)
8 teaspoons of sea salt
1 tablespoon of caraway seeds or fresh or dried dill (OPTIONAL)
1 large container (earthenware crock, glass bowl, or stainless steel cookware)
A cover or plate that fits snugly inside the above container
A brick or stones or any 10-pound weight that's clean
A cloth or towel that will fit over the container

Preparation:
Remove the large, loose outer leaves of the cabbage, rinse them and leave them for later. Core and finely shred the rest of the cabbage. Spread a layer of cabbage (about 1 cup) on the bottom of the container. Sprinkle the layer with a teaspoon of sea salt and a few caraway seeds or dill. Repeat layering with cabbage, salt, and seeds, ending with a layer of salt. Place those loose outer leaves of cabbage over the top layer. Then, press the cabbage down with the plate or cover and place the weight on top of it. Cover the entire container with a cloth or towel and set it aside in a warm place for seven to twelve days, depending on how strong you like your sauerkraut.

After a week or more, remove the weight and the plate. Throw away the leaves on top and skim off the yucky-looking mold from the top layer. Transfer the sauerkraut from the container to glass jars with lids, and refrigerate. It should keep for about a month.

Remedies

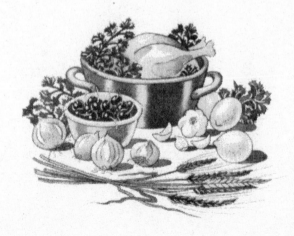

‡ Arthritis (Rheumatism, Bursitis, Gout)

There are many forms of arthritis and rheumatism. And there are many folk remedies that may help heal those conditions, or at least offer relief from them.

You can try more than one remedy at a time. For instance, eat 9 raisins in the morning; have sage tea later in the day; give yourself a ginger/sesame oil rub at night. While you're trying these remedies, pay attention to your body and you'll soon learn what makes you feel better.

THE AMAZING GIN-SOAKED RAISIN REMEDY

Ingredients:
    1 lb. of golden raisins
    Gin (approximately 1 pint)
    Glass bowl (Pyrex is good; crystal is bad)
    Glass jar with lid

Spread the golden raisins evenly on the bottom of the glass bowl and pour enough gin over the raisins to completely cover them. Let them stay that way until all the gin is absorbed by the raisins. It takes about five to seven days, depending on the humidity in your area. (You may want to *lightly* cover the bowl with a paper towel so that dust or flies don't drop in.) To make sure that all of the raisins get their fair share of the gin, occasionally take a spoon and bring the bottom layer of raisins to the top of the bowl and the top to the bottom of the bowl.

As soon as all the gin has been absorbed, transfer the raisins to the jar, put the lid on, and keep it closed. DO NOT REFRIGERATE. Each day, eat 9 raisins. EXACTLY AND ONLY 9 RAISINS A DAY. Most people eat them in the morning with breakfast.

Joe Graedon, author of *The People's Pharmacy*, had the Research Triangle Institute test the gin-soaked raisins for alcohol content. The result: *Less than 1 drop of alcohol was left in 9 raisins. So when people who take the raisins are feeling no pain, it's not because they're drunk, it's because the remedy works.*

Even so, BE SURE TO CHECK WITH YOUR HEALTH PROFESSIONAL TO MAKE SURE THAT THIS REMEDY WILL NOT CONFLICT WITH MEDICATION YOU MAY BE TAKING, OR PRESENT A PROBLEM FOR ANY HEALTH CHALLENGE YOU MAY HAVE, PARTICULARLY AN IRON-OVERLOAD CONDITION.

We've demonstrated this remedy on national television and the feedback has been incredible. One woman wrote to tell us that she had constant pain and no mobility in her neck. Her doctor sent her to several specialists. She spent a fortune, and nothing helped. Her doctor finally told her, "You'll just have to learn to live with the pain." Although that was unacceptable, she just didn't know what to do. And then she saw us on television, talking about a remarkable raisin remedy. We got her letter two weeks after she started the 9 raisins a day. The woman had no pain and total mobility. She also had all of her friends waiting for their gin to be absorbed by their raisins.

This is one of dozens and dozens of success stories we've received. Some people have dramatic results after eating the raisins for less than a week, while it takes others a month or two to get results. There are some people for whom this remedy does nothing. It's inexpensive, easy to do, delicious to eat, and worth a try. Be consistent; eat the raisins every day. Expect a miracle . . . but have patience!

White grape juice is said to absorb the system's acid. Drink 1 glass in the morning and 1 glass before dinner.

If you have morning stiffness caused by arthritis, try sleeping in a sleeping bag. You can sleep *on* your bed, but *in* the zipped-up bag. It's much more effective than an electric blanket because your body heat is evenly distributed and retained. Come morning, there's less pain, making it easier to get going.

Corn silk tea has been known to reduce acid in the system and lessen pain. Steep a handful of the silky strings that grow beneath the husk of corn in a cup of hot water for ten minutes. If it's not fresh-corn season, buy corn silk extract in a health food store; add 10 to 15 drops in 1 cup of water, and drink. Dried corn silk can also be used. Prepare it as you would prepare an herbal tea. You can get dried corn silk at most places that sell dried herbs (see "Sources").

Each of these herbs is known as a pain reducer: sage, rosemary, nettles, and basil. Use any one, two, three, or four of them in the form of tea (see "Preparation Guide"). Have a couple of cups a day, rotating them until you find which makes you feel best.

My friend's grandfather cleared up an arthritic condition and lived to be ninety, following a remedy given to him by a woman who brought it here from Puerto Rico. Squeeze the juice of a large lime into a cup of black coffee and drink it hot first thing each morning. We're not in favor of drinking coffee, but who are we to argue with success?

An old Native American arthritis remedy is a mixture of mashed yucca root and water. Yucca saponin, a steroid derivative of the yucca plant, is a forerunner of cortisone. The side effects of cortisone are too numerous and unpleasant to mention. The side effects of yucca, according to a double-blind study done at a Southern California arthritis clinic, were relief from headaches as well as from gastrointestinal complaints. Sixty percent of the patients taking yucca tablets for that study showed dramatic improvements in their arthritic conditions. While it doesn't work for everyone, it works for a large enough number of people to make it worth a try.

For most people, this remedy is not practical; for many, it's not even possible. Then why take up all this space? The results reported to us were so spectacular that we feel if only one person reads this, follows through, and is relieved of their painful, debilitating condition, it will have been well worth the space on the page.

When we were given this Mexican remedy, we were told that it's for all kinds of "rheumatic" conditions. Some health professionals believe "arthritis" and "rheumatism" are the same, although we could not find a definitive answer. If you're considering trying this remedy, we leave it up to you and your medical consultant to discern whether or not yours is a "rheumatic" condition.

Starting with the first set of directions, you will see why this is usually a "last resort" remedy.

Bring a couple of truckloads of ocean sand to your yard. (What did we tell you?) Select a sheltered spot away from the wind. Dig a hole about 12 feet by 12 feet and about 3 feet deep, then dump the sand in it.

You will, obviously, need help in setting up the above. You will also need help to carry out the treatment. Incidentally, treatment should take place on hot summer days.

Wear a brief bathing suit, lie on your stomach with your face to the side (so you can breathe, of course), and have your body completely covered with sand, except for your head. Stay that way for fifteen minutes. Next, turn over on your back and have your body completely covered with sand, except for your head and face. Have your assistant put sunscreen on your face. Stay that way for fifteen minutes. Then get out of the sandbath, quickly cover yourself with a warm flannel or woolen robe, and head for the shower. Take a hot shower, dry off thoroughly, and go to bed for several hours (three to four) and relax. During all of this, make sure there's no exposure to the wind or to any drafts.

According to an Asian saying: "Rheumatism goes out from the body only through sweating."

During the next couple of hours in bed, you may have to change underwear several times because of profuse sweating. This is good. Be sure to keep rehydrating yourself by drinking lots of water.

One sandbath a day is sufficient. For some people, one week of treatments has been enough to help heal the condition completely.

NOTE: The sandbath must have dry sand and be in your yard, in an area that's sheltered from the wind. The beach is too wet, too breezy, and usually too far from home.

Drink ⅛ teaspoon of cayenne pepper in a glass of water or fruit juice (cherry juice without sugar or preservatives is best). If the pepper is just too strong for you, buy #1 capsules and fill them with cayenne, or you can buy already-prepared cayenne capsules at the health food store. Take two a day.

Combine ½ teaspoon of eucalyptus oil, available at health food stores, with 1 tablespoon of pure olive oil, and massage the mixture into your painful areas.

You may want to alternate the above massage mixture with this one: grate fresh ginger, then squeeze the juice through a piece of cheesecloth. Mix the ginger juice with an equal amount of sesame oil. Massage it on the painful areas. Ginger can be quite strong. If you are uncomfortable from the burning sensation, tone down the ginger by adding more sesame oil to the mixture.

Aloe vera gel is now being used for lots of ailments, including arthritis. You can apply the gel externally to the aching joint and you can take it internally—1 tablespoon in the morning before breakfast and 1 tablespoon before dinner.

Vegetable juices are wonderful for everyone. They can be particularly helpful for arthritis sufferers. Use *fresh* carrot juice as a sweetener with either celery juice or kale juice. (Invest in a juicer or connect with a nearby juice bar.)

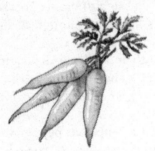

‡ GOUT

Isn't it amazing how much pain you can have from one toe? If you have gout, you probably know it's time to change your diet. The closer you stick to vegetarian cuisine, the faster the gout will go. Okay, eat some fish and lean chicken now and then, but stay away from meat for a while. Also eliminate sugar and white flour from your diet. You may start feeling so good, you may never want to go back to those things.

The one remedy everyone seems to agree on: cherries. Eat them fresh or frozen. Also, drink pure cherry juice daily. You can get pure juice (concentrate) at health food stores.

Soak your gouty foot in comfrey tea (see "Preparation Guide").

A Russian remedy is raw garlic—2 cloves a day. The best way to take raw garlic cloves is to mince them, put them in water (better yet, in cherry juice), and drink them down. No chewing necessary. It doesn't linger on your breath, but it may repeat on you. So does a salami sandwich, and this is a helluva lot healthier.

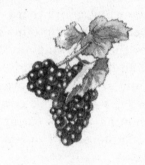

‡ Asthma

Our hearts go out to you asthma sufferers. We've worked especially hard to find effective remedies for this especially troublesome ailment.

We haven't found a sure cure, but we have heard about some remedies that work for some people. While looking for the one that can control your condition, please consult with your health professional every step of the way.

We heard about a man who was able to ease off massive doses of cortisone by using garlic therapy. He started with 1 clove a day, minced, in a couple ounces of orange juice. He gulped it down without chewing any of the little pieces of garlic. That way, he didn't have garlic on his breath. As he increased the number of garlic cloves he ate each day, his doctor decreased the amount of cortisone he was taking. After several months, he was eating 6 to 10 cloves of garlic a day, was completely off cortisone, and was not bothered by asthma.

At the first sign of asthma-type wheezing, saturate two strips of white cloth in white vinegar and wrap them around your wrists, not too tightly. For some people, it stops a full-blown attack from developing.

Generally, dairy products are not good for asthmatics. They're too mucus-forming. We have heard, though, that cheddar cheese might be an exception. It contains "tyramine," an ingredient that seems to help open up the breathing passages.

Cut a 1-ounce stick of licorice (the root, not the candy kind) into slices and steep the slices in a quart of just-boiled water for twenty-four hours. Strain and bottle. At the first sign of a heaviness on the chest, drink a cup of the licorice water. A word of caution, however: Licorice may cause fluid retention and should be used in moderation for people with kidney conditions or high blood pressure.

NOTE (or should we say, WARNING?): In France, licorice water is a drink used by women to give them more sexual vitality.

We were on a radio show when a woman called in and shared her asthma remedy: cherry-bark tea. She buys tea bags in a health food store (if teas are alphabetically listed, it may be under "w" for "wild cherry-bark tea"), and she drinks a cup before each meal and another cup at bedtime. The woman swore to us that it has changed her life. She hasn't had an asthma attack since she started taking it five years ago.

This remedy requires a juicer or a nearby juice bar. Drink equal amounts of endive (also called chicory), celery, and carrot juice. A glass of the juice a day works wonders for some asthmatics.

Remove the eggs from 3 eggshells. Then roast the eggshells for two hours at 400 degrees. The shells will turn light brown. (They'll also smell like rotten eggs.) Pulverize them and mix them into a cup of unsulfured molasses. Take 1 teaspoon before each meal. It just may prevent an asthma condition from acting up.

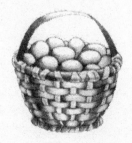

Visualization or mental imagery is a potent tool that can be used to help you heal yourself. Gerald N. Epstein, M.D., director of the Academy of Integrative Medicine and Mental Imagery in New York City (see "Recommended Reading" for his book), suggests that the following visualization be done to stem an asthmatic attack. Do it at the onset of an attack, for three to five minutes. Sit in a comfortable chair and close your eyes. Breathe in and out three times and see yourself in a pine forest. Stand next to a pine tree and breathe in the aromatic fragrance of the pine. As you breathe out, sense this exhalation traveling down through your body and going out through the soles of your feet; see the breath exiting as gray smoke and being buried deep in the earth. Then open your eyes, breathing easily.

NOTE: Learn this visualization and practice it when you're feeling fine so that you know exactly what to do and how to do it the second you feel a wheeze coming on.

Dr. Ray C. Wunderlich, Jr., of the Wunderlich Center for Nutritional Medicine in St. Petersburg, Florida, recommends magnesium for helping take away bronchial spasms. Find a dose of a magnesium preparation that is tolerated (if you get diarrhea, you should cut back on the dosage), and use it to relieve asthma. Do not exceed a total dose of 400 mg of elemental magnesium per day, unless prescribed by a physician.

‡ Back

In our first folk remedy book, we didn't touch on back problems at all, figuring there are almost as many good books on bad backs as there are bad backs. And there are bad backs! It is estimated that eight out of ten people have, at some point in their lives, back pain that disables them. Also estimated is the money spent each year for diagnosis and treatment of back pain—over $5 billion.

Since writing that first book, we've come across some back remedies worth reporting. At best, they'll help; at least, they'll give you something to talk about next time someone tells you his or her back went out.

We are antismoking, so much so that Lydia belongs to an organization that lobbies for nonsmokers' rights. We were happy to find one more reason *not* to smoke—a condition called "smoker's back." According to a study done at the University of Vermont, back pains are more common and more frequent among smokers. They theorize that it has to do with the effect of nicotine on the carbon monoxide levels in the blood, which causes the smoker to cough and the cough, in turn, puts a tremendous strain on the back. Yup! One more good reason to STOP SMOKING! (For suggestions on how to quit, see: "Stop Smoking.")

You need to employ the buddy system for this remedy. Get your buddy to put 20 drops of eucalyptus oil in a tablespoon and warm it by putting a lit match under the spoon for a few seconds. Then have that buddy gently massage the warm oil on your painful area. The "hands on" are as healing as the oil.

Thanks to the guidance of our cousin Linda, who is a physical therapist, the backs of many people who felt that their backs were on the verge of going out, didn't, in fact, go out. If you have had back trouble, you know the feeling we're referring to. When you have that feeling, carefully lie down on the floor, close enough to a sofa or easy chair so that you can bend your knees and rest your legs (knees to feet) on the seat of the sofa or chair. Your thighs should be leaning against the front of the sofa and your tush should be as close as possible, directly in front of it, with the rest of your body flat on the floor. In that position, you're like the start of a staircase. Your body is the lowest step, your thighs are the distance between the steps and your knees-to-feet are the second step. (Did I just confuse you instead of painting a clear picture? Once you're on the floor, it's easy to figure out.)

Stay in that position from fifteen to thirty minutes. It's a restful and healing treatment for the back.

The best and safest way to get up is to roll over on your side, then slowly lift yourself up, letting your arms and shoulders do most of the work.

FOR MEN ONLY: Do you have back or hip pains when you sit for any length of time? Is it something you and your doctor(s) can't quite figure out and so you label it "back trouble"? According to Dr. Elmer Lutz of St. Mary's Hospital in New Jersey, you may need a "wallet-ectomy." If you carry around a thick, bursting-at-the-seams wallet in your hip pocket, it may be putting pressure on the sciatic nerve. Keep your wallet in your jacket pocket and you'll find sitting can be a pleasurable experience.

An Asian remedy for the prevention or relief of lower back problems is black beans, available at supermarkets and health food stores.

Soak a cupful of the black beans (also called *frijoles negros*) overnight. This softens the beans and is said to remove the gas-producing compounds. Then put them in a pot with 3½ cups of water. Bring to a boil, and let simmer for a half hour over low heat. During that half hour, keep removing the grayish foam that forms on top. After a half hour, cover the pot and let it cook for another two hours. If, by the end of that time, there's still water in the pot, spill it out.

Eat 2 to 3 tablespoons of the black beans each day for one month; then every other day for one month.

Fresh beans should be prepared at least every three or four days.

If you need to salt the beans, use a little "tamari"— natural soy sauce available at supermarkets and health food stores.

At the end of two months, if you no longer have lower back pain and you attribute it to the black beans, continue eating them every other day. If you feel your back problem would have healed anyway, stop eating the beans. And, at the first sign of pain in the lower back area, go back to the beans.

Try a flaxseed poultice for chronic back pain. Soak 1 cup of flaxseeds in cold water for ten hours. In an enamel or glass saucepan, bring the mixture to a boil. As soon as they're cool enough to the hand, but still as hot as can be without scalding yourself, make a poultice of the seeds (see "Preparation Guide") and place it on the painful area. You can keep reheating the flaxseeds and reapplying new poultices.

CAUTION: DO NOT APPLY HEAT TO ACUTE BACK PAIN, ONLY TO CHRONIC PAIN. IF YOU HAVE ANY QUESTION

ABOUT WHETHER YOU HAVE CHRONIC OR ACUTE BACK
PAIN, DON'T USE HEAT!

We know a chiropractor who specializes in helping
dancers and athletes. He prescribes vitamin C—500 mg after each meal—to ease the pain and speed the healing of
lower back conditions.

Have you ever had an ice rubdown? The thought of it
sends chills up my spine, but it may help relieve the pain
in that very same area. An easy way to do it is by freezing
a polystyrene cup full of water. Then peel off about a half
inch of the cup's lip and use the rest of the cup as a sort
of knob or handle, gliding the iced surface over your back.
One thing you don't want to do is strain yourself trying to
reach your painful parts, so you may want to ask a friend
to give you the rubdown. Say, you might want to ask a
friend to give you the rubdown even if you don't have back
pain.

‡ Blood Pressure

When blood pressure is measured, there are two numbers reported: the first and higher number is the systolic. It measures the pressure inside the arteries the second the heart beats. The diastolic is the lower number and measures the pressure in the arteries when the heart is at rest.

We saw a woman wearing a T-shirt that said: "Anybody with normal blood pressure these days just isn't paying attention."

More than twenty million Americans have high blood pressure (hypertension). If you're one of those people, obviously you're not alone.

We urge you to take a look at your lifestyle and, once and for all, do something to change whatever is causing the blood pressure problem.

You probably already know the following basics, but in case you need to review them:

- If you're overweight, diet sensibly (without diet pills)
- Eliminate salt (use sea salt in moderation), and cut down or cut out red meat.
- To reduce the stress of your everyday life, try meditation, or some self-help program. Ask a health professional for guidance and reputable contacts.
- If you smoke, stop! (See "Stop Smoking.")
- If you drink, stop! Or at least cut down drastically.

Read on for additional high and low blood pressure health hints.

‡ HIGH BLOOD PRESSURE

Cayenne pepper is a wonderful blood pressure stabilizer.

Add ⅛ teaspoon to a cup of goldenseal tea (see "Preparation Guide") and drink a cup daily.

In a blender, or with a mortar and pestle, crush 2 teaspoons of dried watermelon seeds. Put them in a cup of just-boiled water and let them steep for one hour. Stir, strain, and drink that cupful of watermelon-seed tea a half hour before a meal. Repeat the procedure before each meal, three times a day. After taking the tea for a few days, have your pressure checked and see if it works for you, or if this watermelon remedy is the pits.

Incidentally, watermelon seeds are known to tone up kidney function. Be prepared to use bathroom facilities often. Also, watermelon-seed tea can be bought at health food stores.

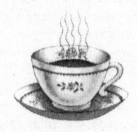

How would you like a hot or cold cup of raspberry-leaf tea? It may help bring down your blood pressure. Combine 1 ounce of raspberry leaves to 2 cups of boiling water and simmer for twenty minutes in an enamel or glass saucepan. Drink 1 cup a day, hot or cold (no ice cubes), and in a week, check the results by having your blood pressure taken.

The faster you talk, the less oxygen you have coming in. The less oxygen, the harder the blood has to work to maintain the supply of oxygen. The harder the blood has to work, the higher the blood pressure seems to go. If that makes sense, please explain it to us. The bottom line here is that if you talk slower, theoretically you will take bigger and better breaths, giving you more oxygen and preventing your blood pressure from climbing.

We've promised our readers, our editor, and ourselves that we wouldn't repeat remedies that were in our first folk remedy book. A promise is a promise, and so we will not talk about garlic, apples, or fish tanks. We will ask that you do yourselves (and us and our publisher) a favor and get a copy of our first *Chicken Soup* book so you can also look into those other effective blood pressure remedies. Thank you!

‡ LOW BLOOD PRESSURE

We heard from a Russian folk healer who recommends drinking ½ cup of raw beet juice when a person feels that his or her blood pressure may be a little too low. This healer also told us that a person with low blood pressure *knows* that feeling.

Deep breathing may bring blood pressure levels up to normal. First thing in the morning and last thing at night, do this breathing exercise: let all the air out of your lungs—exhale, squeezing all the old air out—then let the air in through your nostrils, slowly to the count of seven. When no more air will fit in your lungs, hold tight for the count of fourteen. Next, gently let the air out through your mouth to the count of seven—all the way out. Inhale and exhale this way ten times, twice a day.

Even when your blood pressure is normal, continue this breathing exercise for all kinds of physical benefits.

Licorice root, available at health food stores, will help raise blood pressure. Take it in the morning and at noon. Ebb off when blood pressure is normal.

‡ Body Odor

If you have a problem with bad-smelling armpits, raise your hand. Oops!—better not. Instead, take a shower, then prepare turnip juice. Grate a turnip, squeeze the juice through cheesecloth so that you have 2 teaspoons. *Now* raise your hand and vigorously massage a teaspoon of the turnip juice into each armpit.

A vegetarian friend's sense of smell is so keen, she can stand next to someone and tell whether (s)he is a meat eater. If you are a heavy meat and fowl eater and are troubled by body odor, change your diet. Ease off meat and poultry and force yourself to fill up on green leafy vegetables. There will be a big difference in a short time. You probably won't perspire less, but the smell won't be as strong. That change of diet will be healthier for you in general. And it will be appreciated by all the people in all the crowded elevators you ride.

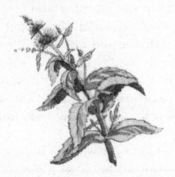

In addition to eating green leafy vegetables, take a 500 mg capsule of wheat grass (powdered juice) daily. Or if your local health food store sells fresh wheat grass juice, have an ounce first thing each morning. Be sure to take it on an empty stomach and drink it down with spring water. The chlorophyll can reduce body odor dramatically or eliminate it completely.

If tension causes you to perspire excessively, which then causes unpleasant body odors, drink sage tea. Use 1½ teaspoons of dried sage, or 2 tea bags in 1 cup of water. Let it steep for ten minutes. Drink it in small doses throughout the day. The tea should help you to relax, so don't sweat it.

‡ Burns

NOTE: When gathering material for the "Burns" section of our first folk remedy book, we called several burn centers throughout the country to make sure we had our facts straight. Although, for the most part, we have not repeated remedies, we feel obligated to repeat this important first-aid information from our other book.

Burns are classified by degrees. A first-degree burn involves painful, red, unbroken skin. A second-degree burn involves painful blisters and broken skin. A third-degree burn destroys underlying tissue as well as surface skin. It may be painless because nerve endings may have also been destroyed. A fourth-degree burn involves deeply charred and blackened areas of the skin.

Second-degree burns that cover an extensive area of skin and all third- and fourth-degree burns require immediate medical attention. Any kind of burn on the face should also receive immediate medical attention as a precaution against swollen breathing passages.

For first-degree burns—grabbing a hot pot handle, grasping the iron side of an iron, the oven door closing on your forearm, a splattering of boiling oil—here are first-aid suggestions using mostly handy household items.

‡ FIRST-DEGREE BURNS

Apply cold water or cold compresses first! Then—

Draw out the heat and pain by applying a slice of raw, unpeeled potato, or a piece of fresh pumpkin pulp, or a slice of raw onion. Leave the potato, pumpkin, or onion on the burn for fifteen minutes, off for five minutes, and put a fresh piece on for another fifteen minutes.

If you burn yourself when there's an uncooked chicken around, place the raw chicken fat directly on the burn or scald. It's said to be extremely soothing.

Puncture either a vitamin E or garlic oil capsule and squeeze the contents directly on the burn.

If you have a smooth piece of charcoal, put it on the burn and keep it there for an hour. Within minutes, the pain may begin to subside.

If you're outdoors, pack mud on the burn to draw out the heat.
Better yet, put your own urine on the burn. The warmth of the fluid will make it radiate with pain for a few seconds, but it will stop soon, and should heal without blistering.

People have had remarkable results with apple cider vinegar. Pour it on the burned or scalded area.

Keep an aloe vera plant in your home. It's like growing a tube of ointment. Break off about a ½-inch piece of stem. Squeeze it so that the juice oozes out onto the burned area. The juice is most effective if the plant is as least two to three years old and the stems have little bumps on the edges.

‡ SECOND-DEGREE BURNS

For at *least* thirty minutes, dip the burned area in cold water. DO NOT USE LARD, BUTTER, OR A SALVE ON THE BURN! Those things seal in the heat and when you get medical attention, the doctor has to wipe off the goo to see the condition of the skin.

If the burn is on an arm or leg, keep the limb raised in the air to help prevent swelling.

‡ CHEMICAL AND ACID BURNS

Until you get medical attention, immediately get the affected area under the closest running water—a sink, a garden hose, or the shower. The running water will help wash the chemicals off the skin. Keep the water running on the burned skin for at least twenty minutes or until medical help arrives.

‡ BURNED TONGUE

Keep rinsing your mouth with cold water. A few drops of vanilla extract on the tongue may relieve the pain.

Ease the pain of a burned tongue by sprinkling some white sugar on it.

‡ ROPE BURNS

Soak the hands in salt water. If salt and water are not available, do as they do in Italy for rope burns: soak the hands in urine.

‡ SUNBURN PREVENTION/SKIN PROTECTION

It's important to protect your skin from the ultraviolet (UV) rays of the sun. Use sunscreen with an SPF (sun protection factor) of at least 15—more is better. Use it all year long, not just in the summer. In fact, during the day, don't leave home without it!

For optimal effectiveness, apply sunscreen a half hour before going outside, allowing it to sink in before you sun out. While you're enjoying the sunny outdoors, reapply sunscreen often, especially if you perspire and/or go swimming. Don't hesitate to slather it on. One ounce of sunscreen should cover the exposed skin of an average-size adult wearing a swimsuit. Yes, you'll probably use up a 4-ounce tube of sunscreen. It's worth it, especially when you consider the cost of down-the-road skin problems.

If you're on medication of some kind, ask your doctor or pharmacist about interactions with sunscreen.

DO NOT use sunscreen on infants six months or younger. The chemicals in it may be too harsh for their delicate skin. Babies that young should never be exposed to the sun for any length of time. The melanin in their skin will not offer them proper protection. When you take a baby out, dress him or her in a tightly woven long-sleeved shirt, long-legged pants, and a wide-brimmed hat.

NOTE: If you have any question about whether or not you can get sunburned, look at your shadow. If your shadow is shorter than your height, you can get sunburned. Don't be surprised to see that your shadow can be shorter than your height as late in the day as 4 P.M. The sun is strongest at about 1 P.M. daylight savings time. If you're going outdoors, be sure to use sunscreen starting at least three hours before and until three hours after 1 P.M.

‡ SUNBURN

When you've gotten more than you've basked for, fill a quart jar with equal parts of milk and ice, and 2 tablespoons of salt. Soak a washcloth in the mixture, wring it out a little, and place it on the sunburned area. Leave it on for about fifteen minutes. Repeat the procedure three to four times throughout the day.

Make a healing lotion by beating the white of an egg and mixing in 1 teaspoon of castor oil. Gently rub it on the sunburned skin.

Or, you may want to empty a package of powdered non-fat milk or a quart of regular low-fat milk into a tub of warm water, and spend the next half hour soaking in it, soothing your sunburn.

NOTE: Severe sunburns can be second-degree burns. If the skin is broken or blistering, treatment should include cold water followed by a dry (preferably sterile) dressing.

‡ SUNBURN PAIN PREVENTION
One way to prevent a sunburn from hurting is by taking a hot—yes hot—shower right after sunbathing. According to a homeopathic principle, the hot water desensitizes the skin.

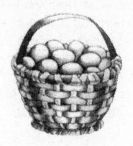

‡ SUNBURNED EYES AND EYELIDS
Make a poultice of grated apples and rest it on your closed eyelids for a relaxing hour.

Make a poultice from the lightly beaten white of an egg (see "Preparation Guide"). Apply the poultice on your closed eyes, secure it in place with an Ace bandage, and leave it on overnight. There should be a big improvement next morning. Cottage cheese in place of egg white is also effective.

‡ Carpal Tunnel Syndrome (CTS)

‡ CARPAL TUNNEL SYNDROME (CTS)

This problem results from swollen tendons that compress the median nerve within the carpal tunnel canal in the wrist. It's usually accompanied by odd sensations, numbness, swelling, soreness, stiffness, weakness, tingling, discomfort, and pain . . . a lot of pain. It's usually caused by continual, rapid use of your fingers, wrists, and/or arms, and many people feel the requirements of their job contribute to the onset of CTS. People who spend their workday at a computer aren't the only ones doing repetitious work: Musicians, supermarket checkers, factory workers, hair stylists, bus drivers, seamstresses, tailors, and countless others are plagued by this repetitive motion injury.

Doctors are recommending vitamin B_6 as a preventative, if you believe that you might become a candidate for CTS because of your job requirements. It's also being used successfully as a treatment. But too much B_6 can be toxic and harmful to the nervous system, so work with your health professional to determine a safe dosage of B_6 for you.

‡ CARPAL TUNNEL CHECKLIST

You may be predisposed to CTS if you are hypothyroid, have diabetes, are pregnant, or if you're on birth control pills. The following items on the checklist are things you can do something about immediately:

- *Do you smoke?* Smoking worsens the condition because nicotine constricts the blood vessels and carbon monoxide replaces oxygen, reducing the blood flow to your tissues.
- *Are you overweight?* Being overweight can present that blood-flow-to-your-tissues problem again. Also, the more weight, the more the muscles must support to move your hand and arm.
- *Do you exercise?* Aerobic exercise—thirty minutes, four times a week—can increase the flow of oxygenated blood to your hands, and help remove waste products from inflammation.

‡ SLEEPING WITH CARPAL TUNNEL

The pain may be more severe while sleeping because of the way you fold your wrist. You may find it more comfortable to wear a splint or wrist brace to bed. Now that the problem is so common, you can get a selection of splints and wrist braces at most drugstores. You may want to wear the splint or brace during the day, too.

If your problem is computer-related, visit your local computer store and see what they have in the way of ergonomic products to support your wrists while at the computer.

‡ EXERCISE FOR CTS PREVENTION

A team of doctors from the American Academy of Orthopedic Surgeons has developed special exercises that can help prevent carpal tunnel syndrome. The exercises, which decrease the median nerve pressure responsible for CTS, should be done at the start of each work shift, as a warm-up exercise, and again after each break.

Stand straight, feet a foot apart, arms outstretched in front of you, palms down. Bring your fingers up, pointing toward the sky. Hold for a count of five. Straighten both wrists and relax the fingers. Make a tight fist with both hands. Then bend both wrists down while keeping the fists. Hold for a count of five. Straighten both wrists and relax the fingers for a count of five. The exercise should be repeated ten times. Then let your arms hang loosely at your sides and shake them for a couple of seconds. *Don't rush through the exercise.* Let the ten cycles take about five minutes.

Dr. James A. Duke, author (see "Recommended Reading") and one of the world's leading authorities on herbal healing traditions, confesses that he uses a computer sometimes as much as fourteen hours a day, but hasn't developed CTS. He gives some of the credit to the fact that he's a man. "Women develop carpal tunnel problems more than men do," explains Dr. Duke, "because the cyclical hormone fluctuations of the menstrual cycle, pregnancy and menopause can contribute to swelling of the tissues that surround the carpal tunnel." Another reason he thinks he's been spared the discomfort of CTS is hand exercises. "Adopting a Chinese technique that improves flexibility," says Dr. Duke, "I hold two steel balls in one hand and roll them around when I'm not typing. The Chinese balls provide a gentle form of exercise, and the rolling motion massages the tiny muscles and ligaments of the hands and wrists." When he's at the computer, he takes frequent breaks to twirl the Chinese balls in each hand.

Chinese balls are inexpensive and readily available at Chinese markets, and some health food stores also carry them.

‡ HERBS FOR CTS

Dr. James Duke in *The Green Pharmacy* (Rodale Press)

reports on quite a few herbs that can help alleviate CTS. With his permission, we share some of them with you:

"Willow bark, the original source of aspirin, contains chemicals (salicylates) that both relieve pain and reduce inflammation. You might also try other herbs rich in salicylates, notably meadowsweet and wintergreen." With any of these herbs, Dr. Duke steeps 1 to 2 teaspoons of dried, powdered bark, or 5 teaspoons of fresh bark, for ten minutes or so, then strains out the plant material. You can add lemonade to mask the bitter taste. Dr. Duke says to drink 3 cups of tea a day. He cautions that if you're allergic to aspirin, you probably shouldn't take aspirin-like herbs.

Chamomile's active compounds (bisabolol, chamazulene, and cyclic esters) also have potent anti-inflammatory action. Dr. Duke says, "If I had CTS, I'd drink several cups of chamomile tea a day."

Dr. Ray Wunderlich, Jr., adds devil's claw and burdock to the list of herbs that often help.

Another way to *Duke* it out is with bromelain, the protein-dissolving (proteolytic) enzyme found in pineapple. According to Dr. Duke, "Naturopaths suggest taking 250 to 1,500 mg of pure bromelain a day, between meals, to treat inflammatory conditions such as CTS. (Bromelain is available at health food stores.)" Since ginger and papaya also contain helpful enzymes, Dr. Duke, who favors food sources to store-bought supplements, suggests, "You might enjoy a Proteolytic CTS Fruit Salad composed of pineapple and papaya and spiced with grated ginger."

One more suggestion from Dr. Duke: "Also known as cayenne, red pepper contains 6 pain-relieving compounds and 7 that are anti-inflammatory. Especially noteworthy is capsaicin. You might add several teaspoons of powdered cayenne to ¼ cup of skin lotion and rub it on your wrists. Or you could make a capsaicin lotion by steeping 5 to 10 red (hot) peppers in 2 pints of rubbing alcohol for a few days. Just wash your hands thoroughly after using any topical capsaicin treatment, as you don't want to get it in your eyes. Also, since some people are quite sensitive to this compound, you should test it on a small area of skin before using it on a larger area. If it seems to irritate your skin, discontinue use."

‡ IF YOU WORK AT A COMPUTER . . .

The National Institute of Occupational Safety and Health recommends that you:

- Position the screen at eye level, about 22 to 26 inches away.
- Sit about arm's length from the terminal. At that distance, the electrical field is almost zero.
- Face forward and keep your neck relaxed.
- Position the keyboard so that elbows are bent at least 90 degrees and you can work without bending your wrists.
- Use a chair that supports your back, lets your feet rest on the floor or on a footrest, and keeps thighs parallel to the floor.
- If you can step away from the computer for fifteen minutes every hour, it can help prevent eyestrain. When you're working at the computer, make a conscious effort to blink often. Frequent blinking will help prevent eye irritation, burning, and/or dry eyes.

‡ Colds, Etc.

‡ COLDS

Soon after we completed our first *Chicken Soup* folk remedy book, the respected Mayo Clinic printed the following in their *Health Letter:*

There is now evidence that our ancestors may have known more about how to treat sniffles than we do. And that should not be surprising. Indeed, scientific study of folk medicines and cures often has proved to be remarkably rewarding.

Moses Maimonides, a twelfth-century Jewish physician and philosopher, reported that chicken soup is an effective medication as well as a tasty food.

A report published in *Chest,* a medical journal for chest specialists, indicates that hot chicken soup is more effective than other hot liquids in clearing mucus particles from the nose. The cause of this beneficial effect is still not fully understood, but the soup does seem to contain a substance which prompts clearing of nasal mucus. And removal of nasal secretions containing viruses and bacteria is an important part of our body's defense against upper respiratory infections. The study gives scientific respectability to the long-standing contention that chicken soup might help relieve a head cold.

Chicken soup—particularly the homemade variety—is a safe, effective treatment for many "self-limiting" illnesses (those not requiring professional attention). It is inexpensive and widely available.

What does it all add up to? Specifically, this recommendation: Next time you come down with a head cold, try hot homemade chicken soup before heading for the pharmacy. We believe chicken soup can be an excellent treatment for uncomplicated head colds and other viral respiratory infections for which antibiotics ordinarily are not helpful. Soup is less expensive and, most significantly, it carries little, if any, risk of allergic reactions or other undesireable side effects.

Have we got a soup recipe for you!

PRESENTING
~ CHICKEN SOUP ~
(THE MEDICINE)

CAUTION: This chicken soup is a *medicine* and is *not* to be eaten as one would eat a portion of soup. Please follow the dosage instructions at the end of the recipe.

Irwin Ziment, M.D., professor of medicine at the University of California School of Medicine, and chief of medicine and director of respiratory therapy at Olive View Medical Center in Los Angeles, is also an authority on pulmonary drugs. Considering the research, experience, and expertise it took to earn his credentials, we believe Dr. Ziment's chicken soup recipe for colds, coughs, and chest congestion should be taken seriously and whenever you have a cold.

DR. ZIMENT'S CHICKEN SOUP

Ingredients:

1 quart homemade chicken broth, or 2 cans low-fat, low-sodium chicken broth

1 garlic head—about 15 cloves, peeled

5 parsley sprigs, minced

6 cilantro sprigs, minced

1 teaspoon lemon pepper

1 teaspoon dried basil, crushed, or 1 tablespoon chopped fresh basil

1 teaspoon curry powder

Optional: hot red pepper flakes to taste, sliced carrots, a
  bay leaf or two

Place all ingredients in a pot without a lid. Bring to a
boil, then simmer for about thirty minutes. (If the soup is
for your own personal use, carefully inhale the fumes during preparation as an additional decongesting treatment.)
Remove the solid garlic cloves and herbs and, along with
a little broth, puree them in a blender or food processor.
Return the puree to the broth and stir. Serve hot.

DOSE: Take 2 tablespoons of Dr. Ziment's Chicken Soup
at the beginning of a meal, one to three times a day. (If
you feel you want a little more than 2 tablespoons, fine,
but do not exceed more than ½ cup at a time.)

Zinc gluconate works wonders for some people. It either
nips the cold in the bud, considerably shortens the duration of the cold, or lessens the severity of it. For it to be
effective, be sure to follow the dosage carefully: Adults,
take 2 lozenges (23 mg each) at the outset and then
1 every two hours thereafter, but not more than twelve
a day, and for no longer than two days. Got it? Also, do
not take them on an empty stomach. Even if you don't feel
like eating, consume half a fruit before you take a lozenge.
Suck on the lozenge so that it comes in prolonged contact with your mouth and throat. Honey-flavored are the
best; lemon are the pits. Zinc gluconate also comes in
46 mg tablets. If you get them instead of the 23 mg, take
1 at the outset and 1 every four hours, not exceeding 6
a day, and for no longer than two days.

For teenage and children's dosages, see the "Infants and
Children" chapter.

NOTE: Some people get stomachaches from zinc.

Respected herbalist Angela Harris says that the combination of echinacea and goldenseal is effective in either

stopping a cold from blossoming, or cutting short the duration and minimizing the severity of a cold. The secret is to take 2 droppers of the extract (available at health food stores) in a few ounces of water every hour for the first four hours of the day you feel a cold coming on. After that, take 2 droppers every four hours. DO NOT take echinacea for more than two weeks at a time. You shouldn't have to.

Another popular remedy, similar to the one above, also for a head cold, is to cut 2 thin-as-can-be strips of orange rind. Roll them up with the white spongy part (the pith) on the outside, and stick one in each nostril. Stay that way until your head cold is better, or you can't stand the rind in your nostrils anymore, whichever comes first. Be sure to leave orange rind sticking out of your nose so you can dislodge it easily.

The first of our five senses to develop is our sense of smell. Eventually, the average human nose can recognize ten thousand different odors, but not when we have a head cold. To clear the head and stop a runny nose, begin by cutting the crust off a piece of bread. Plug in your iron to "hot"—wool or cotton setting. Carefully iron the bread crust. When it starts to burn, lift the iron off the crust and cautiously inhale the smoke through your nostrils for two minutes. Repeat this procedure three times throughout the day. We've been told that the runny nose stops and the head cold clears up in a very short time, one or two days.

Before bedtime, take a ginger bath and sweat away your cold overnight. Put 3 tablespoons of grated ginger in a stocking and knot the stocking closed. (Note: It's easier to grate *frozen* ginger than *fresh* ginger.) Throw it into a hot bath, along with the contents of a 2-ounce container of powdered ginger. Stir the bathwater with a wooden spoon. Then, get in and soak for ten to fifteen minutes. Once you're out of the tub, dry yourself thoroughly, preferably with a rough towel. Put on warm sleep clothes and cover your head with a towel or woolen scarf, leaving just your face exposed. Get in bed under the covers and go to sleep. If you perspire enough to feel uncomfortably wet, change into dry sleepwear during the night.

Talking about "sweating it out" (as we did above), a gem therapist told us that wearing a topaz activates body heat and, therefore, helps cure ailments that may benefit from increased perspiration.

In our first folk remedy book, we talked about the effectiveness of garlic for a cold. The onion, a member of the same family, is also a popular folk medicine for colds. Here are some ways in which the onion is used:

- Cut an onion in half and place 1 half on each side of your bed so you can inhale the fumes as you sleep.
- Eat a whole onion before bedtime in order to break up the cold overnight.
- Dip a slice of raw onion in a glass of hot water. After a few seconds, remove the onion and, when the water cools, start sipping it, and continue to do so throughout the day.
- If you like your onions fried, take the hot fried onions, put them in a flannel or woolen cloth, and bind them on your chest overnight.
- Put slices of raw onion on the soles of your feet, and hold the slices in place with woolen socks. Leave them that way overnight to draw out infection and fever by morning.

* * *

NOTE: If you get colds often, your immune system may need a boost. Check out IMMUNE SYSTEM STRENGTHENER in "Remedies in a Class by Themselves."

‡ FLU

The second you feel fluish, take 1 tablespoon of liquid lecithin (available at health food stores). Continue to take 1 tablespoon every eight hours for the next two days. Some naturalists believe that these large doses of lecithin may prevent a viral flu from flourishing.

This formula was handed down from generation to generation by a family who tells of the many lives it saved during the 1918 flu epidemic in Stuttgart, Germany. They claim that this elixir cleans the harmful bacteria out of the blood.

CAUTION: This remedy is only for people who do *not* have a problem with alcohol.

Peel and cut ½ pound of garlic into small pieces. Put the garlic and 1 quart of cognac (90 proof) in a dark brown bottle. Seal it airtight with paraffin wax or tape. During the day keep the bottle in the sun or other light, warm place, like in the kitchen near the oven. At night move the bottle to a dark, cool place. After fourteen days and nights, open the bottle and strain. Put the strained elixir back in the bottle. It is now ready to be used. The potency of this mixture is said to last one year, so label the bottle with the expiration date accordingly.

If you already have the flu, take 20 drops of the formula with a glass of water, one hour before each meal (three times a day), for five days.

To prevent the flu, take 10 to 15 drops with a glass of water, one hour before each meal, daily during the flu season.

‡ HAY FEVER

March winds bring April showers. April showers bring May flowers. May flowers bring hay fever.

To subdue the symptoms of hay fever, folk medicine practitioners had their patients smoke coffee grounds in a pipe and inhale the smoke.

‡ HAY FEVER PREVENTION

Starting three months before hayfever season, drink 1 cup of fenugreek-seed tea a day. This remedy goes back to the ancient Egyptians and forward to Armenian mountaineers who drink 1 cup of fenugreek tea before each meal to clear and stimulate their senses of smell and taste.

‡ ALLERGIES

There are almost as many types of allergies as there are people who have them. Obviously, allergies need to be handled on an individual basis. We found a few healthful hints that just may help the allergy sufferer:

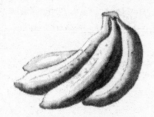

It is said that there are chemicals in bananas that repel allergies—that is, unless you're allergic to bananas. Eat a banana daily.

* * *

Vitamin-rich watercress is said to be an anti-allergen. Eat it in salads, sandwiches, and sauces. It's potent stuff, so eat small portions of it at a time.

We were told that licorice (the herb, not the candy) helps build up an immunity to allergens. Add 3 ounces of cut licorice root (available at health food stores) to 1 quart of water. Boil it for ten minutes in an enamel or glass pot, then strain into a bottle.

DOSE: 1 tablespoon before each meal, every other day until you've taken the licorice-root water for six days. By then, we hope, it will make a difference in terms of your resistance to allergies.

NOTE: Do not take licorice root if you have high blood pressure.

‡ LOOKING FOR A POSSIBLE CAUSE?

We met a woman who has a severe, life-threatening almond allergy. Throughout the nine-month pregnancy, her mother had eaten marzipan on a regular basis. Marzipan is made of almonds. An allergy specialist later told the woman that it's not uncommon for a child to be allergic to a food that the mother craved and ate lots of for months at a time while she was pregnant.

‡ Constipation

You are most likely reading this page because you're seeking a natural laxative. Therefore, you may already know that some of the commercial chemical laxatives can kill friendly bacteria; lessen the absorption of nutrients and get rid of necessary vitamins; stuff up the intestinal walls, turn users into addicts, and eventually *cause* constipation.

We offer easy-to-take, inexpensive, nonchemical constipation relievers that should not present any problem side effects if taken in moderation, using good common sense.

If, after trying these remedies, you still have a persisting problem, you should see a health professional.

Take 2 small beets, scrub them clean, and eat them in the morning. You should have a bowel movement twelve hours later.

Flaxseed is a popular folk treatment for constipation. Take 1 to 2 tablespoons with lots of water right after lunch or dinner. (See "Sensational Six" chapter.)

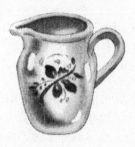

Sunflower seeds are filled with health-giving properties and have also been known to promote regularity. Eat a handful of the shelled, raw, and unsalted seeds every day.

For those of you who feel you need a good colon cleansing, drink an 8-ounce glass of warm sauerkraut juice and then an 8-ounce glass of grapefruit juice (unsweetened)—one right after the other. It should do the job. Okay, so it may rip your throat out in the process.

Eat at least 3 raw fruits a day. One of the 3, preferably an apple, should be eaten two hours after dinner.

We were told about an acupressure technique that is supposed to encourage a complete evacuation of the bowels in fifteen minutes. For three to five minutes, massage the area underneath your lower lip, in the middle of your chin.

The findings of recent studies say that monounsaturated fatty acid—the kind found in olive oil—is best for lowering cholesterol levels. Olive oil is also a help when a laxative is needed. Take 1 tablespoon of extra-virgin, cold-pressed olive oil in the morning and 1 tablespoon an hour after eating dinner.

For some people, brewer's yeast does the trick. Take 1 heaping teaspoon of brewer's yeast and 1 heaping teaspoon of wheat germ with each meal. (Both are available at health food stores.)

Start with small amounts of either or both brewer's yeast and wheat germ. Gradually increase your intake and stop when the amount you're taking works for you.

Are persimmons in season? Try one. It's been known to relieve constipation.

✳   ✳   ✳

For a mild laxative, soak 6 dates in a glass of hot water. When the water is cool, drink it, then eat the dates.

(Also see "Fatigue"—the *figs* remedy.)

‡ Coughs

‡ COUGHS IN GENERAL

Peel and slice a large turnip. Spread honey between all the slices and let it stand for several hours while the turnip/honey syrup oozes out and collects at the bottom of the dish. Whenever the cough acts up, take a teaspoonful of the syrup.

Add ½ cup of raw, shelled, and unsalted sunflower seeds to 5 cups of water and boil in an enamel or glass pot until the water is reduced to about 2 cups. Strain, then stir in ¾ cup of gin and ½ cup of honey. Mix well and bottle it. Whenever the cough acts up, take 1 to 2 teaspoons, but not more than four times a day.

Licorice root contains saponins, natural substances known to break up and loosen mucus. When you have a hacking cough, drink a cup of licorice-root tea (see "Preparation Guide").

NOTE: Do not take licorice root if you have high blood pressure.

An acupressure joint that has been known to stop a cough is the one near the end of the middle finger. With the fingers of your right hand, squeeze the top joint of the left hand's middle finger. Keep squeezing until you stop wheezing.

This bean purée remedy is for one of those mean, down-deep coughs that nothing seems to reach. Put a cupful of kidney beans in a strainer and rinse them with water. Then put them in water and let them soak overnight (while you probably cough your head off, right?). Next morning, drain the beans, tie them up in a clean cloth, and bruise them—

pound them with a blunt object like a rolling pin, frying pan, or hammer. Place the bruised beans in an enamel or glass saucepan with 3 cloves of peeled and minced garlic and 2 cups of water. Bring the mixture to a boil, then simmer for one and a half to two hours, until tender. Add more water if necessary. Take 1 tablespoon of this bean purée the second your cough acts up.

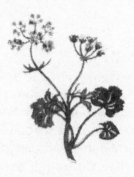

‡ BRONCHIAL COUGHS

Add 3 drops of oil of fennel and 3 drops of oil of anise to 6 tablespoons of honey. Shake vigorously and bottle it. Take 1 teaspoon when you start to cough. If you haven't prepared the syrup in advance of your cough and don't have the necessary ingredients, you may want to settle for second best. Do you have the liqueur called anisette? Take 1 teaspoon of anisette in 1 tablespoon of hot water every three hours.

‡ TICKLING COUGHS

Many people are bothered by a tickling type cough, usually at night in their sleep. Put 2 teaspoons of apple cider vinegar in a glass of water and keep it by your bedside. When the "tickling" wakes you up, swallow one or two mouthfuls of the vinegar water and go back to a restful sleep.

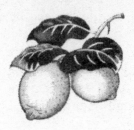

‡ SMOKER'S COUGH

This remedy is updated from the *1888 Universal Cookery Book*. Pour 1 quart of boiling water over 4 tablespoons of whole flaxseed and steep for three hours. Strain, add the juice of 2 lemons, and sweeten with honey (which replaces the crystals of rock candy used in the original remedy). Take a tablespoon when the cough acts up.

An even better remedy for smoker's cough . . . STOP SMOKING! (See "Stop Smoking.")

‡ Diarrhea

Diarrhea is a common condition usually caused by overeating, or a minor bacterial infection, or mild food poisoning, and sometimes by emotional anxiety or extreme fatigue.

Even a quick and simple bout of diarrhea depletes the system of potassium, magnesium, and sometimes sodium, too, often leaving the sufferer tired, dehydrated, and depressed. It's important to keep drinking during and after a siege in order to avoid depletion and dehydration.

NOTE: If diarrhea persists, it may be a symptom of a more serious ailment. Seek professional medical attention.

A West Indian remedy for diarrhea is a pinch of allspice in a cup of warm water or milk. A Pennsylvania Dutch remedy is 2 pinches of cinnamon in a cup of warm milk. A Brazilian remedy calls for 2 pinches of cinnamon and 1 pinch of powdered cloves in a cup of warm milk.

We may as well "milk" this for all it's worth with a Welsh remedy that requires a cup of boiled milk and a red-hot fireplace poker. Carefully place the red-hot poker into the cup of milk. Keep it there for thirty seconds. The poker supposedly charges the milk with iron, which is a homeopathic treatment of diarrhea. Drink the iron-charged milk slowly.

* * *

The combination of cinnamon and cayenne pepper is known to be very effective in tightening the bowels very quickly. In fact, it probably takes longer to prepare the tea than for it to work.

Bring 2 cups of water to a boil, then add ¼ teaspoon of cinnamon and ⅛ teaspoon of cayenne pepper. Let the mixture simmer for twenty minutes. As soon as it's cool enough to drink, have ¼ cupful every half hour.

Add 1 teaspoon of powdered ginger to 1 cup of just-boiled water. To control diarrhea, drink 3 cups of the mixture throughout the day.

Grate an onion and squeeze it through cheesecloth so you get 2 tablespoons (1 ounce) of onion juice. Take the onion juice every hour, along with 1 cup of peppermint tea.

An adsorbent (that's right, *ad*sorbent) substance attaches things to its surface instead of absorbing them into itself. Activated charcoal is the most powerful adsorbent known. Charcoal capsules or tablets can help stop diarrhea quickly by adsorbing the enterobacteria or toxins that may cause the problem. Follow the instructions on the box.

NOTE: Be sure to heed the warning and drug interaction precaution. Activated charcoal is not for everyday use, as it adsorbs the vitamins and minerals you need to be healthy.

If you don't have charcoal tablets or capsules, you might try eating a slice or two of burned (charred) toast.

Raspberry-leaf tea is a popular folk remedy for children and adults. Combine 1 ounce of dried raspberry leaves with 2 cups of water (a piece of cinnamon stick is optional), and simmer in an enamel or glass saucepan for twenty-five minutes. Strain, cool, and drink throughout the day.

*   *   *

According to Hippocrates, the father of medicine, everyone should drink barley water daily to maintain good health.

One of the benefits is its effectiveness in treating diarrhea. Boil 2 ounces of pearled barley in 6 cups of water until there's about one-half the water—3 cups—left in the pot. Strain. If necessary, add honey and lemon to taste. Not only should you drink the barley water throughout the day, you should also eat the barley.

The navel is an acupressure point for treating diarrhea. Using your thumb or the heel of your hand, press in and massage the area in a circular motion for about two minutes.

‡ CHRONIC DIARRHEA

This remedy goes to prove that you can't argue with success. A woman wrote to tell us that Archway Coconut Macaroons—two a day—put an end to her twelve-year bout with diarrhea. She has Crohn's disease, a chronic inflammation of the intestinal wall. Chronic diarrhea is one of the most common and debilitating symptoms of this condition. The woman asked that we include her remedy in our book, hoping it will help others with this problem. Upon further investigation, we found that the People's Pharmacist, Joe Graedon, also reported on these cookies and the success many people had with them. One woman couldn't find the Archway cookies, so she made her own coconut macaroons and they, too, worked like magic. While they don't work for everyone, they may be worth a try. CAUTION: Take into consideration your dietary needs. The cookies are high in fat and contain sweeteners.

‡ DYSENTERY

All of the above "diarrhea" remedies may help treat bacterial dysentery. However, amoebic dysentery (caused by amoebas living in the raw green vegetables of some countries) and viral dysentery are more severe forms of dysentery and should be treated by a health professional.

‡ Ears

‡ EARACHES

An earache may be a sign of a serious infection. The remedies suggested below should not be considered as a substitute for determining the cause of the earache, or for medical treatment.

Also, whenever an ear is draining—discharging thick or thin liquid material from the canal—it may be that the eardrum has ruptured, and that there is a potentially serious infection. If that's the case, get medical attention immediately.

There are times when you have an earache and can determine that medical care is not required at that moment. It is only at such times that you should consider the following remedies:

Fill the ear with 3 warm (not too hot) drops of olive oil and plug the ear with a puff of cotton. Do this three or four times a day until the earache is gone.

This remedy is a little more complex but might provide faster relief than the one above. Mix the juice from grated fresh ginger with an equal amount of sesame oil. Drop in 3 drops of the mixture and plug the ear with a puff of cotton. Keep it there for a few hours.

* * *

This reflexology remedy requires something sterile and hard to bite down on. The ideal thing is one of those cotton cylinders the dentist uses. What we do is wad up a piece of cheesecloth and it works fine. Place the wad of whatever in back of the last tooth on the side of the aching ear, and bite down on it for five minutes. This stimulates the pressure point that goes directly to the ear. Repeat this procedure every two hours until the earache is gone. This acupressure process relieves the pain of an earache and has been known to improve hearing as well.

Another effective way of easing the pain of an earache is with a soothing chamomile poultice (see "Preparation Guide"). If you don't have the loose herb, use a couple of tea bags instead.

Cut a large onion in half. Take out the inside of the onion so that the remaining part will fit over your ear. Warm the onion "earmuff" in the oven, then put it over your ear. Be sure it's not too hot. It should help draw out the pain.

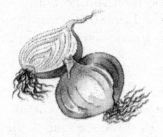

‡ RUNNY EAR INFECTION
You'll need to go to a good, old-fashioned Italian fish store for this remedy. Get the soft, transparent bone from a squid. Bake it until it turns black and crush it into a powder. Taken orally, ½ teaspoon before breakfast and another ½ teaspoon before dinner, it is said to help clear up a runny ear infection.

‡ "SWIMMER'S EAR" PREVENTION

A lot of people seem to be plagued by recurrent, painful ear canal infections soon after swimming. Here's a solution that may prevent infections: Add 1 teaspoon of white vinegar to 4 tablespoons (2 ounces) of just-boiled water. Once the liquid is cool, store it in a bottle. Right after swimming put 2 drops of the vinegar mixture in each ear. Plug each ear with a cotton puff and stay that way for about ten minutes.

‡ GETTING THE WAX OUT

Wax buildup? Warm 2 teaspoons of sesame oil and put a spoon in each ear. Be sure the oil is not too hot. Gently plug the ear with a puff of cotton, and allow the oil to float around for a while. Once the sesame oil softens the wax, you can wash out the ears completely. The results: no more oil, no more wax.

‡ EARLOBE INFECTION

Men as well as women have been troubled with earlobe infections from ear-piercing. Put castor oil on your lobes a few times a day—the more the better. The infection should clear up in two or three days at most. If it gets worse, seek professional help.

‡ RINGING (TINNITUS)

We heard about a woman who had constant ringing in her ears for years. None of the specialists could help her. As a last resort, she started using castor oil. After a month, the ringing subsided considerably. Within three months, it was completely gone.

If your ringing or buzzing is not caused by medication you're taking, and if your doctor doesn't know what it's from or what to do for it, you might want to try castor oil—3 or 4 drops a day in each ear. To get full benefit from the castor oil, plug the ear with cotton once you've put in the drops, and keep it there overnight.

In a blender, combine 6 large, peeled garlic cloves and 1 cup of almond oil or extra virgin, cold-pressed olive oil. Blend until the garlic is finely minced. Clean a glass jar by pouring just-boiled water into it. Once the jar is dry, pour the garlic and oil mixture into the jar, put the cover on, and refrigerate it for seven days. Then strain the liquid from the jar into a clean eyedropper bottle. At bedtime, take the chill out of a small amount of the liquid, then put 3 drops in each ear and plug the ears with cotton puffs. Remove the cotton in the morning. Chances are, if the ringing is going to stop, it will do so within two weeks.

Always keep this preparation refrigerated, and do not keep it longer than a month.

‡ PARTIAL LOSS OF HEARING

A loud noise, a cold, or wax buildup can cause partial loss of hearing. In Sicily, where garlic is a cure-all, they stew a few cloves in olive oil, then press it and strain it. On a daily basis, 3 or 4 drops of the garlic/olive oil juice are placed in the ear(s) and plugged up with cotton. It is said to restore one's hearing.

"Hey, I can hear now."
"Good. I've been wanting to tell you something: YOU SMELL OF GARLIC!"

‡ IMPROVE YOUR HEARING

Aerobic exercise, including brisk walking or bicycling, can help prevent some age-related deterioration in the ears, as well as damage caused by exposure to loud noises. Exercise also increases the ability to hear faint sounds. This good news comes from results of studies conducted at Miami University of Ohio—you heard right, Miami U. of Ohio—which concluded that aerobic exercise improves hearing by circulating blood to inner ear cells and bringing them more oxygen and an increased supply of chemicals that prevent damage to them.

‡ Emphysema

If you've been diagnosed as having the lung condition known as emphysema, and you're still smoking cigarettes, don't bother reading this anymore. Turn to the "Stop Smoking" chapter. Come back when you've stopped smoking.

Now then, combine ½ teaspoon of raw honey with 5 drops of anise oil and take this dosage a half hour before each meal.

We've heard positive reports about this remedy. It's worth a try.

When you're having a hard time breathing, sit down, lean forward, and put your elbows on your knees. This position can make breathing easier because it elevates the diaphragm, the most important muscle used for breathing.

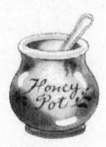

See "Lung Power" in the "Remedies in a Class by Themselves" chapter and consider learning to play the harmonica.

‡ Eyes

‡ CINDERS

When something gets in your eye, try not to rub the eye. You'll irritate it, then it's hard to tell whether or not the foreign particle is out.

Get a tissue ready. With one hand pull your lashes so that the upper lid is away from your eye. With the other hand, appropriately position the tissue in the center of your face and blow your nose three times.

If the remedy above didn't work for you and you have access to a kitchen, put some pure olive oil in a teaspoon, hold a lit match under it for a few seconds—long enough to *slightly* warm the oil. Then put 2 drops in the eye that has the particle. What? You don't have an eyedropper? Buy one at any health food store or pharmacy and keep it in your medicine chest for just such occasions.

NOTE: If you put olive oil, or anything else that's helpful for your eyes, in an eyedropper bottle, label it properly and immediately. Then, before using it, carefully check to be sure you're not putting some toxic substance in your eyes.

Until you get an eyedropper for the above remedy, you may want to try this: 1 drop of fresh lemon juice (1 drop only!) in 1 ounce of warm water and wash your eye with it. It should remove the particle and it is surprisingly soothing.

NOTE: To get the most benefit from eyedrops, keep your eyes closed for about two minutes after putting in the drops. That will prevent the blinking process from pumping the drops out of your eyes.

‡ IRRITATIONS

If your eyes are irritated from a foreign particle, cooking fumes, cigarette smoke, dust, etc., put 2 drops of castor oil in each eye, or 2 drops of milk in each eye.

Use any of the "Eyewashes" listed at the end of this chapter.

‡ BLOODSHOT EYES

If you don't drink in excess and you get enough sleep, but still have bloodshot eyes on a regular basis, you may be bothered by your contacts, allergic to the eye makeup you wear, or you may be deficient in vitamin B_2 (riboflavin). Take 15 mg of B_2 daily. You might also want to have a tablespoon of brewer's yeast every day.

Use any of the "Eyewashes" listed at the end of this chapter, and you might want to try the grated potato remedy listed under "Black Eye."

‡ STIES

Roasted-bancha tea bags are available at most health food stores. Steep a tea bag in hot water for ten minutes and add 1 teaspoon of sea salt (available at health food stores as well as supermarkets). Saturate a cotton pad in the lukewarm liquid and apply it to your closed eye, keeping it there for ten minutes at a time, three times a day.

❊   ❊   ❊

In addition to, or instead of, the above remedy, dab on some castor oil several times throughout the day until the sty disappears.

‡ STY PREVENTION

Lydia went to school with a girl named Madeline whose nickname was "Sty." She always seemed to have a sty coming or going. If you're like Madeline and are prone to sties, prepare a strong cup of burdock-seed tea every morning and take 1 tablespoon before each meal and 1 at bedtime.

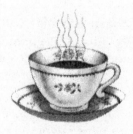

‡ CATARACTS

There are amazing new surgical procedures now for removing cataracts. Know your options. While you're investigating the alternatives, you might want to try one of the following:

Honey! No, we're not getting overly friendly here, we're just relaying a remedy to help clear away a cataract.

Every day for two weeks, put a drop of raw honey in the eye with the cataract. It will sting like crazy until the tears wash away the pain. At the end of the two weeks, if you "see" an improvement, continue the daily regime for another two weeks. Then have your eye doctor confirm the improvement.

Dr. Gladys of the Association for Research and Enlightenment Clinic of Phoenix, Arizona, recommends 2 drops of castor oil in each eye at bedtime. If there is no improvement after a month, try another remedy.

NOTE FOR USING EYEDROPS: To get the most benefit from eyedrops, gently pull out your lower lid and let the liquid drop into the eye pocket. Then keep your eyes closed for about two minutes after putting in the drops. That will prevent the blinking process from pumping the drops out of your eyes.

Noted English physician Nicholas Culpeper was a great believer in the healing effects of chamomile eyewashes to improve a cataract condition. (See "Eyewashes" at the end of this chapter.)

Research scientists have found that a deficiency of vitamin B_2 (riboflavin) can cause cataracts. Tests done at the University of Georgia Hospital have built a most impressive case for B_2 preventing cataracts as well as clearing up existing conditions. Brewer's yeast is the source richest in riboflavin. Take 1 tablespoon a day and/or 15 mg of vitamin B_2. Along with a B_2 vitamin, take a B-complex vitamin to avoid high urinary losses of B vitamins.

‡ CATARACT PREVENTION
See the above vitamin B_2 remedy.

‡ EYESTRAIN (TIRED EYES)
If your eyes are strained and tired, chances are the rest of your body is also dragging. Lie down with your feet raised

higher than your head. Relax that way for about fifteen minutes. This gravity-reversing process should make you and your eyes feel refreshed and rarin' to go.

Cut 2 thin slices of a raw red potato and keep them on your closed eyelids for at least twenty minutes. Red potatoes are said to have strong healing energy, but any other potato will work, too.

Steep rosemary in hot water for ten minutes. (That line sounds like a recipe for a soap opera.) Use a rosemary tea bag or 1 teaspoon of the loose herb in a cup of just-boiled water. Saturate a cotton pad with the tea and keep it on your eyes for fifteen minutes. Rosemary should help draw out that tired-eye feeling.

Also, see "Palming"—the last remedy under "Vision Improvers."

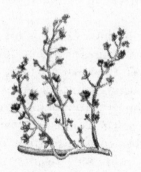

‡ EYESTRAIN PREVENTION

Looking at red ink on white paper for long periods of time can cause eyestrain and headaches. Stay out of the red!

‡ DRY EYES

Tear ducts that do not produce enough fluid to keep the eyes moist can result in an uncomfortable *dry eye* condition that is characterized by irritation, burning, and a gravelly feeling.

If you use artificial tears, DO NOT use any product that also "gets the red out." When your eyes are red or bloodshot, it's because there's a problem. Your body's way of handling the problem is by enlarging the delicate veins or blood vessels in your eyes. The eye drops that "get the red out" are vasoconstrictors that shrink those veins so that you don't see them. This is not a good thing and is only a temporary masking of the problem. Also, your eyes can become dependent on those drops and, when you stop using them, the problem will worsen and the blood vessels in your eyes will be more dilated than before.

Also, make sure the box says *preservative-free* or *nonpreserved*. Preservatives in artificial tears can be harmful to your eyes.

Check out homeopathic eye drops for dry eye syndrome. Homeopathic medications are without side effects and are well tolerated by even the most sensitive system. They work to restore health rather than to suppress symptoms. Similasan Eye Drops, known throughout Europe, are now available here in America. The company provides samples of the drops for eye doctors to give to their patients. For information, including impressive results of a Harvard study, call Similasan at: 1-800-426-1644.

You may be able to eliminate artificial tears completely by adding omega-3 fatty acids to your diet, which may increase the viscosity of oils made by the body, mostly in the skin and eyes. Omega-3 is found abundantly in cold-water fish and flaxseed oil. This means eating several servings of fish a week—all varieties of salmon (except smoked) and canned white tuna—and/or taking flax oil. We suggest you read about the many benefits of flax oil in our "Sensational Six" chapter. CAUTION: If you're on blood-thinning medication, or have uncontrolled high blood pressure or bleeding disorders, or are going in for surgery, be sure to check with your doctor before taking flax oil.

Help your eyes do the work they're supposed to do by opening the clogged oil glands in the eyelids. Take a warm, white washcloth and place it on your closed eyelids. Leave it on until it turns cool—five to ten minutes. Do this a few times a day—obviously, the more the better.

‡ DRY EYE DON'TS

Don't use a blow dryer on your hair unless you absolutely have to.

Don't go outdoors without sunglasses. The wraparound kind are excellent for keeping the wind out.

Don't dry out your eyes with heating or cooling systems in your home, office, car, and even on an airplane. Keep the heat or air-conditioning to a minimum or turn off completely unless it's really necessary. And then, be sure the vents are not pointing in your direction.

Don't go for any length of time without blinking. People at computers have this problem. Every time you click the mouse, blink. Every time you save a document, blink. Every time you swallow, blink. Do whatever it takes to make yourself conscious of blinking often, especially when you're sitting in front of the computer.

Don't wear contact lenses all the time.

Don't smoke. One more reason not to smoke is that the smoke adds to the burning and other dry eye symptoms.

Don't cry about it. It makes the problem worse. Tears brought on by emotion wash away the oils that prevent dry eyes.

‡ BLACK EYE

Pour witch hazel on a cotton pad and apply it to the bruised, closed eye. Lie down with your feet slightly higher than your head for a half hour while the witch hazel stays in place.

Walk into a door, did you? I hope it was the door to the kitchen. If you're there now, peel and grate a potato (a red potato is best). Make a poultice out of it (see "Preparation Guide") and keep it on the black eye for twenty minutes. Potassium chloride is one of the most effective healing compounds, and potatoes are the best source of potassium chloride.

This remedy is also beneficial for bloodshot eyes.

‡ EYE TWITCH

Pressure and tension can cause eyelid twitching. Aside from the two-week vacation you should take, eat calcium-rich foods. According to some nutritionists, adults can and should get all the calcium we require through nondairy foods: green vegetables, sesame seeds, whole grains, unrefined cereals, canned salmon and sardines, soy milk, and other soy products including tofu.

‡ INFLAMED EYES AND EYELIDS

Crush a tablespoon of fennel seeds and add it to a pint of just-boiled water. Let it steep for fifteen minutes, then dunk cotton pads in the liquid and place them over your eyelids for about fifteen minutes.

There's an herb called horsetail (see "Sources" for vendors who might sell the herb). Steep 1 teaspoon of dried horsetail in hot water for ten minutes. Saturate cotton pads with it and apply the pads to your eyelids for ten minutes.

Redunk the pads in the liquid, then keep them on your eyes for another ten minutes. One more time! After half an hour, the inflammation should start calming down.

Freshly sliced cucumber on eyelids for about fifteen minutes is soothing and healing. You may also peel the cucumber and squeeze a couple of drops of juice directly into each eye.

Also, use any of the "Eyewashes" listed at the end of this chapter. Try "Palming," too. It's the last remedy under "Vision Improvers."

‡ CONJUNCTIVITIS (PINKEYE)
The plant eyebright is particularly effective in the treatment of conjunctivitis. Add 3 drops of tincture of eyebright (available at health food stores) to a tablespoon of boiled water. When cool enough to use, bathe the eye in the mixture. Since this condition is a contagious one, wash the eye cup thoroughly after you've washed one eye, then mix a new batch of eyebright with water and wash the other eye. Do this three or four times a day until the condition clears up. Or, use the "Eyewashes" listed at the end of this chapter.

Goat milk yogurt can help clear up this uncomfortable condition. Apply a yogurt poultice (see "Preparation Guide") to the infected eye(s) daily. Also, eat a portion or two of the yogurt each day. The active culture in yogurt can help destroy the infection-causing bacteria in your system.

‡ NIGHT BLINDNESS
Since this remedy seems so yucky, we would not have included it had we not heard of the wonderful results from several reliable sources. Every day for two weeks, put a drop

of raw honey in each eye. (We said "yucky" didn't we?) It stings like crazy for a few seconds until tears wash away the pain. Within a week or two there should be a noticeable improvement in your night vision.

Try "Palming." It's the last remedy under "Vision Improvers."

‡ SUN BLINDNESS

Sun blindness is caused by exposure to large expanses of snow or ice for a considerable length of time. For this condition, make a poultice from the lightly beaten white of an egg. Bandage the poultice on the closed eyes and sleep that way. There should be a big improvement next morning. Cottage cheese in place of egg white is also effective.

‡ SUN BLINDNESS PREVENTION

Skiers will find this remedy most helpful in coping with large expanses of snow. Eat a handful of sunflower seeds every day. (Buy them shelled, raw, and unsalted.) Within no time, the eyes may have a much easier time adjusting to the brightness of the snow, thanks to the sunflower seeds . . . and a good pair of sunglasses or goggles.

‡ VISION IMPROVERS

You know all the talk about carrots being good for your eyes? They are! Drink 5 to 6 ounces of fresh carrot juice twice a day for at least two weeks. Obviously, you'll need a juicer or a nearby juice bar. After the two weeks, ease off to one glass of carrot juice a day . . . forever!

NOTE: If you have a candida/yeast problem, skip the carrot juice because of its high sugar content.

❈   ❈   ❈

According to J. I. Rodale, founder of *Prevention* magazine, sunflower seeds are a miracle food. We agree. Eat a handful (shelled, raw, and unsalted) every day.

We've heard that wearing a gold earring in your left ear improves and preserves one's eyesight. We weren't going to include this as a remedy because we thought it's a useless superstition. Then we read in David Louis's book, *2201 Fascinating Facts*, that pirates believed that piercing their ears and wearing earrings improved their eyesight—and the swashbucklers may have been right. The idea, which had been scoffed at for centuries, has been reevaluated in light of recent acupuncture theory, which holds that the point of the lobe where the ear is pierced is the same acupuncture point that controls the eyes.

Hmmmm. Get out the gold earrings.

We've thoroughly researched "palming" and no two of our resources agree on the procedure. We'll give you a couple of variations. Test them and see what works for you.

Sit. (They all agree on that.) Rub your hands together until you feel heat. With your elbows on the table, place the heels of your hands over your eyes, blocking out all light. Some feel it's better to keep one's eyes open in the dark; others advocate closed eyes. The length of time to sit this way also ranges—from two minutes to ten minutes.

Eyes opened or closed, any length of time, "palming" is beneficial for improving vision, for nearsightedness, tired eyes, astigmatisms, inflammations, and may even help squinters stop squinting.

‡ GLAUCOMA

NOTE: Glaucoma is a serious condition. When using any home remedy, be sure it's done under the supervision of an eye specialist.

Vitamin B_2 (riboflavin) deficiency is one of the most common vitamin deficiencies in this country. It's also the vitamin that's most beneficial for eye problems such as glaucoma. Take 100 mg daily, along with a B-complex. The reason for the B complex is that large doses of any one of the B vitamins can result in urinary losses of other B vitamins.

Bathe the eyes morning and evening in an eyewash made with fennel seed, chamomile, or eyebright. (See "Eyewash Directions" for instructions on using these eyewashes.)

‡ EYEWASH DIRECTIONS

REMINDER: Always remove contact lenses before doing an eyewash.

You'll need an eye cup (available at drugstores). Carefully pour just-boiled water over the cup to clean it. Without contaminating the rim or inside surfaces of the cup, fill it half full with whichever eyewash you've selected. Apply the cup tightly to the eye to prevent spillage, then tilt your head backward. Open your eyelid wide and rotate your eyeball to thoroughly wash the eye. Use the same procedure with the other eye.

‡ EYEWASHES

Commercial eyedrops eliminate the redness because of a decongestant that constricts the blood vessels. Using these drops on a regular basis can worsen the problem. The blood vessels will enlarge again in less and less time. Make your own eyedrops from the following herbs, or just bathe your eyes with these eyewashes:

‡ Eyebright

To make an eyebright eyewash, add 1 ounce of the whole, dried herb, eyebright, to 1 pint of just-boiled water and let it steep for ten minutes. Strain the mixture thoroughly through a superfine strainer or through unbleached muslin. Wait until it's cool enough to use.

Or, add 3 drops of tincture of eyebright to a tablespoon of boiled water, and, again, wait until it's cool enough to use.

‡ Chamomile

Add 1 teaspoon of dried chamomile flowers to 1 cup of just-boiled water. Steep for five minutes and strain the mixture thoroughly through a superfine strainer or through unbleached muslin. Wait until it's cool enough to use.

Or, add 12 drops of tincture of chamomile to 1 cup of just-boiled water.

‡ Fennel Seeds

Add 1 teaspoon of crushed fennel seeds to 1 cup of just-boiled water. Steep for five minutes and strain the mixture thoroughly through a superfine strainer or through unbleached muslin. Wait until it's cool enough to use.

‡ Sunburned Eyes and Eyelids (See: "Burns.")

‡ EYEGLASS CLEANERS

To avoid streaks on your eyeglass lenses, clean them with a touch of vinegar or vodka.

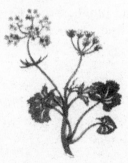

‡ Fainting Prevention

When you feel as though you're going to faint, sit down and put your head between your knees. If you're in an appropriate place, lie down with your feet and torso elevated so that your head is lower than your heart. That's the secret of preventing a faint—getting your head lower than your heart so the blood can rush to your brain.

In India, instead of smelling salts people take a couple of strong whiffs of half an onion to bring them around.

If it's a scorcher of a day and you're feeling every degree of it, or if you're in a very warm room that's making you feel faint, just run cold tap water over the insides of your wrists. If there are ice cubes around, rub them on your wrists. Relief is almost immediate.

A friend of ours is a paramedic. When one of her patients is about to faint, she pinches the patient's philtrum—the fleshy part between the upper lip and nose. That prevents the faint from happening.

Check your eating habits. Are you eating regularly at mealtimes? Are you eating good, wholesome meals with a sufficient amount of protein, and without an excess of sweets and refined foods?

* * *

CAUTION: If you faint and don't know why, consult a doctor. Fainting can be a symptom of an ailment that needs medical treatment.

‡ Fatigue

‡ PICKER-UPPERS

A Chinese theory is that "tiredness" collects on the insides of one's elbows and the backs of one's knees. Wake up your body by slap-slap-slapping both those areas.

Tough day at the office? Need to get that second wind? Ready for a drink? Tired of all these questions? Add 1 tablespoon of blackstrap molasses to a glass of milk (regular, skim, soy, or rice milk) and bottoms up.

Call on your imagination for this visualization exercise. Sit up with your arms over your head and your palms facing the ceiling. With your right hand, pluck a fistful of vitality out of the air. Next, let your left hand grab its share. Open both hands, allowing all that energy to flow down your arms to your neck, shoulders, and chest. Start over again. This time, when you open your hands, let the energy flow straight down to your waist, hips, thighs, legs, feet, and toes. There! You've revitalized your body. Now stand up feeling refreshed.

A bunch of grapes can give you a bunch of energy. Hey, maybe that's why you always see pictures of people eating grapes at those bacchanalian orgies.

Grapes may be too perishable for you to carry around, but dried figs aren't. And they sure can pack an energy punch. They're delicious, satisfying, have more potassium than bananas, more calcium than milk, have a very high dietary fiber content, and they have no cholesterol, fat, or sodium. Most important, figs have easily digestible, natural, slow-burning sugars that will get you going and keep you going, unlike the quick-fix, fast-crash processed sugar in junk food. Herbalist Lalitha Thomas, who lists figs as one of the *10 Essential Foods* (in her book of the same name), says to make a serious effort to get *unsulfured* figs. Eat a few at a time—but don't overdo it. Figs are known to help prevent or relieve constipation.

When you just can't keep your eyes open or your head up and you don't know how you'll make it to the end of the day at your office, run away from it all. Go to the bathroom or a secluded spot and run in place. Run for two minutes and it should help you keep going the rest of the day.

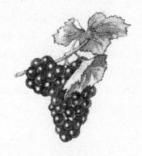

‡ STAMINA

Three cheers for chia. According to a study of American Indians, a pinch of chia seeds helped the braves brave their arduous round-the-clock days of hunting. Ground chia seeds, available at health food stores, can be sprinkled on salads or in soup for those on-the-go-around-the-clock days when stamina counts.

‡ START YOUR DAY
THE ENERGY WAY

Here's how to wake up your metabolism in the morning: into a glass squeeze the juice of half a grapefruit.

Fill the rest of the glass with warm water. Drink it down slowly, then eat the fruit of the squeezed-out half grapefruit. Now that your thyroid is activated, have a productive day!

If, after a full night's sleep, you get up feeling sluggish, it may be due to a tired liver. Stand up. Place your right hand above your waist, on the bottom of your ribs on your right side, with your fingers apart, pointing toward your left side. Place your left hand the same way on your left side. Ready? You press your right hand in, then back in place. You press your left hand in, then back in place. You do the Hokey-Pokey and you turn your— No! Sorry, I got carried away. Now then, press your right hand in, then back in place. Press your left hand in, then back in place. Do it a dozen times on each side when you get up each morning. In a couple of weeks, this liver massage may make a big difference in your daily energy level. Cutting out heavy starches and sweets from your diet can also go a long way in adding to your get-up-and-go.

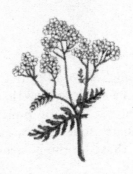

‡ MENTAL ALERTNESS

We've read case histories in which, within weeks, the intake of bee pollen not only increased a person's physical energy, but restored mental alertness and eliminated lapses of memory and confusion. Suggested dosage: 1 teaspoon of the granular bee pollen after breakfast, or two 500 mg bee pollen pills after breakfast. (Read all about bee pollen in the "Sensational Six Superfoods" chapter.)

Start by taking just a few granules of bee pollen a day to make sure you have no allergic reaction to it. If all is well after three days, increase the amount to a quarter teaspoon. Gradually, over the next month or two, work your way up to 3 teaspoons of bee pollen throughout each day.

‡ Feet, Ankles, and Legs

"Ow! Do my shoes hurt me!"
"No wonder your shoes hurt you. You have them on the wrong feet."
"But I don't have any other feet."

There's wisdom in that silly joke. We *don't* have any other feet. That's why we should take care of the ones we have.

According to podiatrist Dr. Steven Baff, 40 percent of American children develop foot ailments by age six and, by adulthood, 80 percent of Americans suffer from foot problems.

CAUTION: If you have circulation problems, or diabetes, do not use any of these remedies without the approval and supervision of your health professional.

‡ CORNS

Make a paste out of 1 teaspoon of brewer's yeast and a few drops of lemon juice. Spread the mixture on a cotton pad and apply it to the corn, binding it in place and leaving it overnight. Change the dressing daily until the corn is gone.

A paste of powdered chalk and water should also take care of the corn.

A Hawaiian medicine man recommends pure papaya juice on a cotton pad, or a piece of papaya pulp directly on the corn. Bind in place and leave it on overnight. Change daily until the corn is gone.

Australian shepherds squeeze the juice from the stems of dandelions and apply it to the corn every day until the corn disappears, usually within a week.

‡ TIRED, SORE, BURNING—
OH, YOUR ACHING FEET!

This remedy requires 2 basins or dishpans or 4 plastic shoe boxes. Fill 1 basin or 2 shoe boxes with ½ cup Epsom salts and about 1 gallon of hot (not scalding) water; fill the other basin or the other 2 shoe boxes with ice cubes. Sit down with a watch or timer. Put your feet in the hot water for one minute and then in the ice cubes for half a minute. Alternate back and forth for about 10 minutes. Your feet will feel better. This procedure also helps regulate high blood pressure and may prevent varicose veins, improve circulation, and, if done on a regular basis, relieve chronic "cold feet."

A modified version of the above is: Stand in the bathtub and first let hot water run on your feet, then let ice cold water run on your feet, timing it the same as above.

DO NOT EXCEED ONE (1) MINUTE OF HOT OR COLD WATER ON YOUR FEET!

Add 1 cup of apple cider vinegar to a basin or 2 plastic shoe boxes filled halfway with lukewarm water. Then soak your feet in it for at least fifteen minutes. The heat and hurt should be gone by then.

Boil or roast a large turnip until it's nice and soft. Then mash it and spread half of it on a white cotton handkerchief; spread the other half on another handkerchief. Apply the turnip mush to the bottoms of your bare feet, bandage them in place, and sit with your feet elevated for about half an hour. This sole food should draw out the pain and tiredness.

‡ SWEATY FEET

The average pair of feet gives off about ½ pint of perspiration daily. It's amazing we don't all seem to slosh around. Well, for those of you who feel like you do . . .

Put some bran or uncooked oat flakes into your socks. It should absorb the sweat and make you feel more comfortable. Start conservatively, with about 1 tablespoon. Add more if needed.

‡ ATHLETE'S FOOT

Grate an onion and squeeze it through cheesecloth to get onion juice. Massage the juice into the fungus-infected areas of your foot. Leave it on for ten minutes, then rinse your foot in lukewarm water and dry it thoroughly. Repeat this procedure three times a day until the condition clears up.

NOTE: To avoid reinfecting yourself with athlete's foot, soak your socks and hose in vinegar. Also wipe out your shoes with vinegar. The smell of vinegar will vanish (say that three times fast) after being exposed to the air for about fifteen minutes.

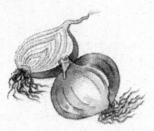

‡ CALLUSES

You can soften your calluses by applying any of the following oils: wheat germ oil, castor oil, sesame seed oil, or olive oil. Apply the oil as often as possible throughout the day, day after day.

❊   ❊   ❊

Walking barefoot in the sand, particularly wet sand, is wonderful for your feet. It acts as an abrasive and sloughs off dead skin that could lead to corns and calluses.

If you're not near the beach for the above remedy, add 1 tablespoon of baking soda to a basin or to 2 plastic shoe boxes filled halfway with lukewarm water and soak your feet in it for fifteen minutes. Then take a pumice stone (available at health food stores and pharmacies) and carefully file away the tough skin.

Cut an onion in half (the size of the onion should be determined by the size of the callused area the onion's cut surface has to cover). Let the onion halves soak in wine vinegar for four hours. Then take the onion halves and apply them to the calluses. Bind them in place with plastic wrap, put on socks, and leave them overnight. Next morning, you should be able to scrape away the calluses. Don't forget to rinse your feet to get the onion/vinegar smell off.

‡ ROUGH AND CRACKED HEELS

Before bedtime, wash your feet with warm water and dry them. Liberally apply petroleum jelly on your feet, massaging it into the rough and cracked areas. Wrap each foot with plastic wrap. Put socks on and sleep that way. Repeat the process nightly until your feet are fine. It shouldn't take more than a week . . . probably a lot less.

‡ TOES—TINGLING AND NUMBNESS

Daily doses of vitamin B_6 and B complex have been known to eliminate tingling and numbness in toes. Take 100 to 200 mg B_6. Check the amount of B_6 in the B complex, and make sure you are taking *less* than 300 mg B_6 daily. Too much B_6 can be toxic.

‡ INGROWN TOENAIL

We were surprised to learn that a tendency toward ingrown toenails is inherited.

If you have an ingrown toenail, relieve the pain with a footbath. In a plastic shoe box, add ½ ounce of comfrey root (available at health food stores) to ½ gallon (2 quarts) of warm water. Soak your foot in it for twenty minutes.

Once the nail is softened from soaking, take a piece of absorbent cotton and twist it so that it's like a thick strand of thread. Or you can twist together a few strands of unwaxed dental floss. Gently wedge the "thread" under the corner of the nail. That should prevent the nail from cutting into the skin. Replace the strands a couple of times a day, every day, until the nail grows out.

The nail should be cut straight across, not down into the corners, and not shorter than the toe. You might want a podiatrist to trim the toenail properly. Pay careful attention so you'll be able to take care of your toes yourself and avoid another ingrown nail (and another podiatrist bill).

‡ WEAK ANKLES

This exercise will promote toe flexibility and strengthen the arches as well as the ankles.

Get a dozen marbles and a plastic cup. Put them all on the floor. Pick up each marble with the toes of your right foot and, one by one, drop them in the cup. Then do the same with the toes of your left foot. You may want to add to the fun by timing yourself and seeing if you can keep breaking your previous record. Whatever happens, try not to lose your marbles.

Each night, right before bed, take a raw oyster in the palm of your hand and rub your ankle with it until it just about disintegrates. Then take another raw oyster in the palm of your hand and rub the other ankle. This is supposed to strengthen one's ankles. Why else would you do such a silly thing?

‡ LEG CRAMPS

After doing our homework, we've learned that leg cramps can be caused by a variety of nutritional deficiencies. For instance, magnesium, potassium, vitamin E, calcium, or protein. Are you eating lots of greens? (We don't mean *two* olives in your martini.) Cut down on fatty meats, sugar, and white flour. In a week, see if there's a difference in the incidence of leg-cramping.

If you take a diuretic, you may be losing too much potassium from your system, which may be causing leg cramps. If that's the case, eat a banana or two every day. You might also want to ask your doctor to take you off the chemical diuretic and find a natural one, like cucumber, celery, or lettuce.

Organic Consumer Report says that muscular cramps that usually occur at night can be relieved within twenty minutes by taking this combination: 1 tablespoon of calcium lactate, 1 teaspoon of apple cider vinegar, and 1 teaspoon of honey in half a glass of warm water.

Vermont's noted doctor D. C. Jarvis has a remedy similar to the one above. He suggests 2 teaspoons of honey at each meal, or honey combined with 2 teaspoons of apple cider vinegar in a glass of water before each meal as a way to prevent muscle cramps.

Before you get out of bed in the morning, turn yourself around so that you can put your feet against the wall, higher than your body. Stay that way for ten minutes. Do the same thing at night, right before you go to sleep. It will improve blood circulation and may prevent muscle cramps. It's also an excellent *stretch* that in itself may prevent cramps.

Lancet, the British medical journal, reports that vitamin E is helpful in relieving cramps in the legs. Take 100 I.U. of vitamin E before each meal, daily. Within a week or two there should be a positive difference.

Take advantage of the therapeutic value of a rocking chair. Rock whenever you watch television and for at least one hour before bedtime. For those of you who sit most of the time, a rocking chair may prevent varicose veins and blood clots, and improve circulation as well as relieve you of leg cramps.

Drink 1 cup of red raspberry-leaf tea in the morning and 1 cup at night. Do this every day and you may no longer have leg cramp attacks.

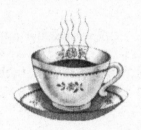

According to Dr. John M. Ellis, three weeks after prescribing vitamin B_6 to his patients suffering from leg cramps, they were no longer bothered by them. The B_6 also took care of numb and tingling toes. Take 100 to 200 mg of B_6 along with a B complex. Check the amount of B_6 in the B complex. Make sure it does NOT exceed 300 mg B_6. Too much B_6 can be toxic.

* * *

We were told about a simple technique called "acupinch." It's an acupressure procedure that may help relieve the pain of muscle cramps almost instantly. The second you get a cramp, use your thumb and your index finger and pinch your philtrum—the skin between your upper lip and your nose. Keep pinching for about twenty seconds. The pain and cramp should disappear.

Try drinking an 8-ounce glass of water before bedtime.

‡ JOGGER'S LEG CRAMP PREVENTION

After your run, find a cool stream of moving water in which to soak for fifteen to twenty minutes. For those of you who can only dream of that, every night, right before going to bed, walk in about 6 inches of cold water in your bathtub for about three minutes. The feedback from runners who do this has been very convincing that the cold water walks do prevent leg cramps.

Be sure to have those nonslip stick-ons on the floor of the tub.

‡ Female Problems

We've come a long way, baby!

Today, we talk openly about menstruation, pregnancy, and menopause, not as sicknesses, but as natural stages of life. We also recognize and deal with premenstrual tension and menopausal irregularities.

We are finally learning to question the male-dominated medical profession after hearing countless stories about hysterectomies, radical mastectomies, and other surgery that's sometimes performed whether a woman needs it or not.

Knowledge is power. Television talk shows, bookstores, local libraries, and the Internet are filled with women's health information. Take advantage of these sources so that you can take responsibility for your own body and good health by intelligently choosing the most appropriate medical care and caregivers.

Meanwhile, here are some home remedies *whispered* down from generation to generation.

‡ MENSTRUATION: LIGHTEN THE FLOW

To lighten an unusually heavy menstrual flow, drink yarrow tea—2 to 3 cups a day until the period is over. To prepare the tea, add 1 or 2 teaspoons of dried yarrow (depending on how strong you want the tea to be) to 1 cup of just-boiled water. Let it steep for ten minutes. Strain and drink. You may not like the taste of the tea, but so what, as long as you get results.

‡ MENSTRUAL CRAMPS

Reduce your salt intake the week before you're expecting your period. It should cut down on the cramps and the bloating.

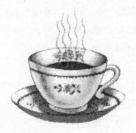

When it comes to menstrual cramps, how do naturalists spell relief? L-e-a-f-y g-r-e-e-n-s. Eat lots of lettuce, cabbage, and parsley before and during your period. To get the full benefit of all vegetables, eat them raw or steamed. Aside from helping reduce cramps, the leafy greens are diuretics and will relieve you of some bloat.

When your menstrual pains drive you to drink, make that drink an ounce or two of warm gin. Gin is prepared from a mash consisting of 85 percent corn, 12 percent malt, and 3 percent rye, and is distilled in the presence of juniper berries, coriander seeds, etc. Go easy on the gin. You may get rid of the cramps, but you don't want to have to deal with a hangover. And obviously, don't follow this remedy if you have a problem or a past history of problems with alcohol. If you do try this remedy, don't drive!

‡ MENSTRUAL IRREGULARITIES

On a daily basis, thoroughly chew then swallow 1 tablespoon of sesame seeds. Or grind flaxseeds and sprinkle a tablespoon on your cereal, soup, or salad. Both have been known to regulate menstrual cycles.

‡ MORNING SICKNESS

A doctor at Brigham Young University recommends 2 or 3 capsules of powdered ginger first thing in the morning to avoid morning sickness.

This folk remedy is an oldie and a goodie. Mix ⅓ cup of lime juice and ⅛ teaspoon of cinnamon in ½ cup of warm water. (It sounds like it could bring on morning sickness.) Drink it as soon as you awaken. It's really known to be quite effective.

‡ QUICK LABOR, EASY DELIVERY, AND SPEEDY RECOVERY ("WHO COULD ASK FOR ANYTHING MORE?")

Many sources agree on raspberry tea for the mother-to-be. What our sources don't agree on is when to start drinking the tea. Some say right after conception; others, three months before delivery; and still others, six weeks before the due date.

The consensus is that pregnant women should drink 2 to 3 cups of raspberry tea a day, starting *at least* six weeks before the expected birth. Ask your obstetrician about it.

Add 1 teaspoon of dried raspberry leaves to 1 cup of just-boiled water. Let it steep for five minutes, strain, and drink.

See the SEX chapter—For Women Only—"Muscle Strengthener," which will tell you about a way to strengthen your bladder control, as well as the bladder control section that appears later in this chapter.

‡ BREAST-FEEDING

To stimulate milk secretion, drink a mixture of fennel seeds and barley water. Crush 2 tablespoons of fennel seeds and simmer them in a quart of barley water (see "Preparation Guide") for twenty minutes. Let it cool and drink it throughout the day.

Peppermint tea is said to increase the supply of mother's milk and it's also known to relieve nervous tension and improve digestion. Drink 2 to 3 cups a day.

Add lentil soup to your diet. Lentils are very rich in calcium and other nutrients necessary for nursing mothers.

‡ MENOPAUSE

If you are getting hot flashes, it could mean one of two things: either the paparazzi are following you, or you're going through menopause. We have no remedy for the paparazzi, but we can report on three recommendations that have been known to relieve some of the menopausal chaos.

Step into a tub that has 6 inches of cold water in it. Carefully, walk back and forth for about three minutes. Be sure to have nonslip stick-ons on the floor of the tub. Step out, dry the feet thoroughly, and put on a pair of walking shoes (socks are optional), and take a walk—even if it's just around your room—for another three minutes.

Andrew Weil, M.D., the guru of integrative medicine, has an effective recommendation for hot flashes and other symptoms of menopause. It is a combination of 3 herbs (all readily available at herb and health food stores): dong quai, chaste tree (Vitex), and damiana. Take 2 capsules or 1 dropper of each of these herbs (you can mix the three herbal extracts into a cup of warm water) once a day at noon. Continue this regimen until the hot flashes stop, then taper it off gradually.

Naturalists call pure licorice and sarsaparilla "hormone foods." Use the two of them as teas and drink them often (see "Preparation Guide").

NOTE: If you're on medication, do not take herbs unless you check with your health professionals.

‡ CYSTITIS

Women who frequently get cystitis should empty their bladders, if passion allows, *before* intercourse. It's also possible to lessen the number of attacks or stop them forever by passing water immediately *after* intercourse.

Forgo oral sex.

We've heard folk remedies requiring the cystitis sufferer to take baths. Recently, we were told by a research scientist that baths may cause the recurrence of the condition. If you are a bath-taker and have recurring cystitis, refrain from taking a bath for at least a month, and shower instead. You just may find you aren't troubled with cystitis anymore.

According to Native Americans, corn silk (the silky strands beneath the husk of corn) is a cure-all for urinary problems. The most desirable corn silk is from young corns, gathered before the silk turns brown. Take a handful of corn silk and steep it in 3 cups of boiled water for five minutes. Strain and drink the 3 cups throughout the day. Corn silk can be stored in a glass jar, not refrigerated. If you can't get corn silk, use corn silk extract, available at health food stores. Add 10 to 15 drops of the extract to a cup of hot water. Dried corn silk is also available.

‡ BLADDER CONTROL

The Kegel or pubococcygeus exercises can help you gain control over your bladder, strengthen your abdominal muscles, and tighten muscles that can enhance sexual activity.

Each time you urinate, start and stop as many times as possible. While squeezing the muscle that stops the flow of urine, pull in on the muscles of the abdomen. You can also do this exercise when *not* urinating. Sit at your desk, in your car, at the movies—anyplace—and flex, release, flex, release.

For another suggestion, see the SEX chapter—For Women Only—"Muscle Strengthener."

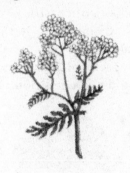

‡ Gallbladder

The gallbladder is the liver's companion and assistant. Its job is to store bile produced by the liver, then release it to dissolve fats. Your job is to keep the gallbladder healthy and functioning. These remedies may help.

The most popular folk remedy for the gallbladder is black radish. Juice the radish either with a juice extractor or by grating the radish and squeezing it through cheesecloth. Take 1 to 2 tablespoons of black radish juice before each meal. Do it for two weeks or more. Your digestion should improve and so should the condition of your gallbladder.

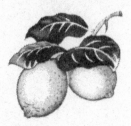

An inflamed, irritated, or clogged gallbladder can make you feel sluggish and tired, even when you first wake up in the morning. Take 3 tablespoons of fresh lemon juice in half a glass of warm water, a half hour before breakfast. Try this for one week and see if there's a difference in your morning energy level. Lemon juice is known to stimulate and cleanse the gallbladder.

If you have had gallbladder surgery, you may help the healing process with peppermint tea—1 cup one hour after eating each of the two biggest meals of the day. Menthol, the active ingredient in peppermint, gives the liver and gallbladder a workout by stimulating bile secretion.

‡ Hair

Human hair is almost impossible to destroy. Other than its vulnerability to fire, it cannot be destroyed by changes of climate, water, or other natural forces. When you think of the ways some of us abuse our hair with bleaches, dyes, rubber bands, permanents, mousses, sprays, and that greasy kid stuff, you can see how resistant it is to all kinds of corrosive chemicals. No wonder it's always clogging up sinks and drainpipes.

While hair may not be *destroyed* by the abuse mentioned above, it may look lifeless and become unmanageable and unhealthy.

One way to tell whether or not hair is healthy is by its stretchability. A strand of adult hair should be able to stretch to 25 percent of its length without breaking. If it's less elastic than that, it's less than healthy.

‡ BAD HAIR DAYS

If your self-esteem is in the cellar and you're feeling less than confident, capable, or sociable, it may be because you're having a bad hair day. The findings of a Yale University study confirmed the negative effect of a crummy coif on the psyche. The fascinating aspect of the study was that *men* were more likely to feel less smart and less capable than *women* when their hair stuck out, was badly cut, or was otherwise mussed up.

Here are remedies to help you have healthy hair, be the best tressed person around, and boost your self-esteem.

‡ SHAMPOO/TREATMENT FOR CORRECTING AND PREVENTING PROBLEMS

This treatment is said to clean, condition, and give a shine to the hair. It should also help get rid of dandruff and nourish the scalp and hair. If it does only half of what it promises, it's worth doing. All you need is:

1 egg yolk and ½ cup warm water for thin and short hair
2 egg yolks and 1 cup warm water for average shoulder-length hair
3 egg yolks and 1½ cups warm water for thick and long hair

Combine and beat the egg yolk(s) and water thoroughly. Massage the mixture into your scalp and on every strand of hair. To make sure the entire head of hair is saturated and fed this protein potion, massage for five minutes, then put a plastic bag over your scalp and hair for another five minutes. Next, rinse with tepid water (hot water will cook the egg, making it difficult to remove). When you're sure that all of the egg is out of your hair, rinse one more time.

Use this as a maintenance shampoo once or twice a month to help prevent problems from returning.

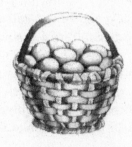

‡ CONDITIONER FOR WISPY HAIR

This conditioning treatment comes highly recommended for taming flyaway hair. (If you don't know what we mean, you don't have it.) Beat an egg into 2 ounces (6 tablespoons) of plain yogurt. After shampooing your hair, vigorously rub this mixture into the scalp and hair for three minutes. Wrap a towel around your hair and leave it that way for ten minutes. Rinse with tepid water. If this treatment works for your hair, repeat the procedure after every shampooing.

‡ DRY SHAMPOO

If your building is having plumbing problems, or your city is having a water shortage, or you just don't feel like washing your hair, you can dry-shampoo it with cornmeal or cornstarch. Sprinkle some on your hair. Put a piece of cheesecloth or already-run panty hose on the bristles of a hairbrush and brush your hair with it. The cornmeal/cornstarch will pull out the dust from your hair; the cloth will absorb the grease.

Complete the job with a silk scarf. Shine your hair with it, using it as you would a buffing cloth on shoes. After a few minutes of this, if your hair doesn't look clean and shiny, tie the scarf around your head and no one will know the difference.

Coarse or kosher salt is known to be an effective dry shampoo. Put 1 tablespoon of the salt in silver foil and in the oven to warm for five minutes. Using your fingers, work the warm salt into the scalp and throughout the hair. As soon as you feel that the salt has had a chance to absorb the grease and dislodge the dust, patiently brush it out of your hair. Wash the brush thoroughly, or use an already-clean brush and brush again to make sure all the salt has been removed.

NOTE: Do not use table salt. Not only will you still have dirty hair, but it will look as though you have dandruff, too.

‡ SETTING LOTIONS

Don't throw away beer that's gone flat. Instead, dip your comb in it, comb it through your hair, and you have a wonderful setting lotion. Incidentally, the smell of beer seems to disappear quickly.

A friend of ours is a professional model and she knows many tricks of her trade. Her favorite hair-setting lotion is fresh lemon juice. The hair takes longer to dry with the juice on it, but the setting stays in a lot longer. When she runs out of lemons, she uses the bottled lemon juice in the fridge and that works well, too.

If beer or lemon aren't your cup of tea, try milk. Dissolve 4 tablespoons of skim milk powder in 1 cup of tepid water. Use it as you would any commercial hair-setting lotion. Unlike most commercial products, the milk helps nourish the scalp and hair.

‡ DANDRUFF

Massage 4 tablespoons of warm corn oil into your scalp. Wrap a warm, wet towel around your head and leave it there on the corn oil for half an hour. Shampoo and rinse. Repeat this treatment once a week.

This treatment is for dandruff and other scalp problems. Grate a piece of ginger and squeeze it through cheesecloth, collecting the juice. Then mix the ginger juice with an equal amount of sesame oil. Rub the ginger/sesame lotion on the entire scalp, cover the head with a sleep cap or wrap a dish towel around the head, and sleep with it on. In the morning, wash with an herbal shampoo (available at most stores where shampoo is sold), and the final rinse should be with 1 tablespoon of apple cider vinegar in 1 quart of warm water. Repeat this treatment three or four times a week until the dandruff or other scalp problems vanish.

Prepare chive tea by adding 1 tablespoon of fresh chives to 1 cup of just-boiled water. Cover and let it steep for twenty minutes. Strain and, making sure it's cool, rinse your hair with it right after you shampoo.

You many also want to consider using the first remedy in this chapter—"Shampoo/Treatment for Correcting and Preventing Problems."

‡ ENERGIZING HAIR ROOTS

According to reflexology expert Mildred Carter, "To energize the hair roots, grab handsful of hair and yank gently. Do this over the whole head. This is also said to help a hangover, indigestion, and other complaints. To further stimulate these reflexes in the head, lightly close your hands into loose fists. With a loose wrist action, lightly pound the whole head. This will not only stimulate the hair, but also the brain, bladder, liver, and other organs."

The reflexologist believes that tapping the reflexes in the head with a wire brush can add even greater electrical stimulation to the hair as well as other parts of the body.

‡ STOPPING HAIR LOSS AND PROMOTING HAIR GROWTH

In an average lifetime, the hair on the head grows about twenty-five feet.

Each of us loses about a hundred hairs a day from our

scalp. Mostly, the hairs grow back. When they don't, the hairstyle changes from "parted" or "unparted," to "departed."

Ninety percent of baldness can be attributed to hereditary factors. Can something be done to prevent it or overcome it? The people who gave us these remedies say, "Yes!"

An Asian remedy to stop excessive amounts of hair from falling out is sesame oil. Rub it on your scalp every night. Cover your head with a sleep cap, or wrap a dish towel around it. In the morning, wash with an herbal shampoo (available at most stores where shampoo is sold). Your final rinse should be with 1 tablespoon of apple cider vinegar in 1 quart of warm water.

Another version of the above nightly/daily treatment calls for equal amounts of olive oil and oil of rosemary. Combine the two in a bottle and shake vigorously. Then massage it into the scalp, cover the head, sleep, awaken, shampoo, and rinse, same as above.

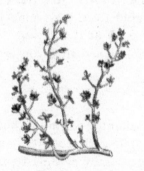

Yet another version of the above nightly/daily procedure—garlic oil. Puncture a couple of garlic pearls, squish out all the oil and massage it into your scalp. Then follow the aforementioned routine of covering the head overnight and, in the morning, be sure to shampoo and rinse.

* * *

And still another version of these massage scalp remedies: Take half of a raw onion and massage the scalp with it. It's known to be an effective stimulant. Cover the head overnight and shampoo and rinse in the morning.

Just this one more hair-restoring/baldness-preventing formula. A man who recently emigrated to the United States from Russia told us that many barbers in the former Soviet Union recommend this to their customers. Combine 1 tablespoon of honey with 1 jigger of vodka and the juice from a medium-size onion. Rub the mixture into the scalp every night, cover, sleep, awaken, shampoo, and rinse, as described in the first of this series of remedies.

We heard that Rodney Dangerfield came up with a formula: alum and persimmon juice. It doesn't grow hair. It shrinks your head to fit what hair you've got.

‡ "NATURAL" HAIR COLORING

Herbal or vegetable dyes take time because the color must accumulate. Look at it this way, if you get the gray out gradually, no one will realize you ever had any gray to begin with.

‡ Brunettes

We have 2 hair-darkening formulas, both with dried sage, which adds life to hair and prevents dandruff.

Prepare dark sage tea by adding 4 tablespoons of dried sage to 2 cups of just-boiled water and letting it steep for two hours. Strain. This dark tea alone will darken gray hair, but for a stronger hair color, add 2 cups of bay rum and 2 tablespoons of glycerine (available at pharmacies). Bottle this mixture and don't forget to label it. Every night, apply the potion to your hair, starting at the roots and working your way down. Stop the applications when your hair is as dark as you want it to be.

Or, if you're a teetotaler and don't want to use the rum, combine 2 tablespoons of dried sage with 2 tablespoons of black tea and simmer in 1 quart of water for twenty minutes. Let it steep for four hours, then strain and bottle. Massage it into your hair daily until your hair is the color of your choice. When you need a touch-up, mix a fresh batch of the teas.

Taking sesame-seed tea internally has been known to darken one's hair. Crush 2 teaspoons of the sesame seeds and bring to a boil in 1 cup of water. Then let it simmer for twenty minutes. As soon as it's cool enough to drink, drink it, seeds and all. Have 2 to 3 cups daily and keep checking the mirror for darkening hair.

Add a little life to your hair color right after you shampoo by pouring a cool cup of espresso through your hair. Let it stay there for five minutes and rinse.

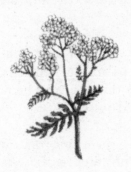

‡ *Blondes*

Dried chamomile can help add golden highlights to wishy-washy blond hair. Add 4 tablespoons of dried chamomile to 2 cups of just-boiled water and let it steep for two hours.

Strain and use it as a rinse. Be sure to have a basin set up so you can catch the chamomile and use it over again for the next two or three shampoos.

As with most herbal rinses, you mustn't expect dramatic results overnight, if ever. Chamomile tea, no matter how strong you make it, will not cover black roots.

That reminds us of something we've wondered about for a while. In Sweden, are there brunettes with blond roots?

Squeeze the juice out of two big lemons, strain, and dilute with 1 cup of warm water. Comb the juice through your hair. Be very careful not to get any of it on your skin. Why? Because you should sit in the sun for fifteen minutes in order to give your hair the glow of a summer day. If your skin has lemon juice on it, it can cause a burn and give your skin mottled stains.

After the sunbath, rinse your hair thoroughly with warm water, or better yet, with chamomile tea.

NOTE: Be sure your skin is properly protected in the sun with sunscreen of at least 15 SPF (higher is better).

‡ Redheads

Add radiance to your red hair right after you shampoo by pouring a cup of strong Red Zinger tea (available at health food stores) through your hair. Let it remain there for five minutes and rinse.

Juice a raw beet (in a juice extractor) and add three times the amount of water as there is juice. Use this as a rinse after shampooing.

NOTE: Since there are many shades of red, we suggest you do a test patch with the beet juice to see how it reacts on your specific color.

‡ *Gray, Gray, Go Away!*

Many vitamin therapists have seen proof positive that taking PABA (para-aminobenzoic acid)—300 mg a day—plus a good B-complex vitamin, also daily, can help change hair back to its original color over a period of two months or more.

We got this suggestion from a nutritionist who doesn't have one gray hair on his head. (Of course, he's only twelve years old.)

In a glass of water, mix 2 tablespoons of each of the following: apple cider vinegar, raw unheated honey, and blackstrap molasses. Drink this mixture first thing in the morning. Not only should it help you get rid of gray hair, but it should also give you a lot more energy than people who haven't gotten gray yet.

‡ HELPFUL HAIR HINTS

‡ *Prevent Gray from Yellowing*

By adding a couple of teaspoons of laundry bluing to a quart of warm water and using it as your final rinse after shampooing, you can prevent gray hair from turning that yucky yellow.

‡ *Green-Hair-from-Pool Treatment*

Chlorinated pool water can turn a bleached blonde into the not-so-jolly "green" giant. Dissolve 6 aspirins in a pint of warm water, massage it into your wet hair, and the green will never be seen. Rinse thoroughly with clear water. Ho! Ho! Ho!

‡ *No-No Number 1: Rubber Bands*

We've always been told not to wear rubber bands in our hair. We just found an explanation for it: The rubber insulates the hair and stops the normal flow of static electricity, so hair elasticity is reduced and the hair breaks more easily.

‡ No-No Number 2: Combing Wet Hair

Combing wet hair stretches it out, causing it to be less elastic and break more easily.

‡ Attention Parents: Gum Remover

To remove gum from hair without doing a Delilah, take a glob of peanut butter, put it on the gummed area, then rub the gum and peanut butter between your fingers until the gum is on its way out. Use a comb to finish the job, then get that careless kid under the faucet for a good shampooing.

‡ A Permanent's Pungent Odor Remover

The distinctive smell of a permanent has a habit of lingering. Tomato juice to the rescue! Saturate your dry hair with tomato juice. Cover your hair and scalp with a plastic bag and stay that way for ten minutes. Rinse hair thoroughly, then shampoo and rinse again.

‡ Hair Spray Remover

In the middle of shampooing, massage 1 tablespoon of baking soda into your soaped-up hair. Rinse thoroughly. The baking soda should remove all the hair spray buildup.

‡ Improvised Setting Rollers

If you have long hair and want to experiment setting it with big rollers, try used frozen juice cans, opened at both ends.

‡ Grounding Your Hair

When static electricity makes your hair temporarily unmanageable, you might want to zap it with static spray used on records.

Or, rub a sheet of fabric softener on your hair as well as on your brush or comb.

For chronic wispy hair condition, see "Conditioner for Wispy Hair" earlier in this chapter.

‡ Hangovers

Have a hangover? Feel like pulling your hair out? Good idea, but don't go all the way. Just pull your hair, clump by clump, until it hurts a little. According to a noted reflexologist, hair-pulling is stimulating to the entire body and can help lessen the symptoms of a hangover.

When you have a hangover headache, eat a raw persimmon for relief. From now on, if you insist on drinking, make sure it's persimmon season.

Hangover sufferers are often advised to "sleep it off." That's smart advice, since a contributing factor to hangovers is the lack of REM (rapid eye movement) sleep which alcohol seems to suppress. So, yes, sleep it off!

A Chinese hangover remedy calls for eating 10 strawberries and drinking a glass of fresh tangerine juice. Sounds good even if you don't have a hangover.

Hungarian Gypsies recommend a bowl of chicken soup with rice. What could be bad?
Cysteine is an amino acid which helps the body manufacture glutathione, which is an antioxidant that gets depleted when it has the chore of contending with alcohol. According to a recent study at the University of California, cysteine is present in chicken. Therefore, chicken soup may help replenish the body's needed supply of cysteine, easing hangover symptoms at the same time.

A glass of sauerkraut juice is said to be effective. If the pure juice is hard for you to take, add some tomato juice to it. Or, eat lots of raw cabbage. That's been known to work wonders.

If you've overindulged and are anticipating waking up in the morning with a hangover, take a vitamin B complex with 2 or 3 glasses of water before you go to bed. If you pass out before remembering to take the B complex, when you awaken with your hangover take the vitamin as soon as possible.

Some of the B-complex vitamins are B_1 (thiamine), B_2 (riboflavin), nicotinamide, and pyridoxine. They are helpful in aiding: carbohydrate metabolizing, nerve functioning, the cellular oxidation process, and the dilation of blood vessels, all helpful for hangovers. Impressed?

We were on a radio show in Boston and an Irishman called in, identifying himself that way, to share his hangover remedy—the only one that works for him every time: bagel, cream cheese, and lox (smoked salmon). He discovered this sure-cure after marrying a Jewish woman who served him the sandwich one morning-after-the-night-before, as a typical Sunday brunch.

There are some of you who will not be happy until you find a "hair of the dog" hangover remedy. Here's one we were told comes from a voodoo practitioner in New Orleans: in a blender, add 1 ounce of Pernod, 1 ounce of white crème de cacao, and 3 ounces of milk, plus 3 ice cubes. Blend, drink, and good luck!

‡ SOBERING UP

This is a Siberian method of sobering up a tippler. Have him lie flat on his back. Place the palms of your hands on his ears. Next, rub both ears briskly and strongly in a circular motion. Within minutes, the person should start coming around. While he may be a lot more sober than before you rubbed his ears, he should not be trusted behind the wheel of a car.

FACT: For every ounce of alcohol you drink, it takes an hour to regain full driving faculties. In other words, if you have 4 ounces of alcohol by 8 P.M., you should not drive until at least midnight. Actually, we don't think it's a good idea to drive at all on the same night you've done any drinking. Statistics can bear that out.

‡ INTOXICATION PREVENTION

We're reporting the remedies that supposedly prevent one from getting drunk, but we ask that you please take full responsibility for your drinking. If you drink, do not trust or test your reflexes—especially behind the wheel of a car—no matter how sober you seem to feel, or which preventive remedies you take.

Native Americans recommend 6 raw (not roasted) almonds before drinking.

This remedy comes from healers in West Africa. They suggest eating peanut butter before imbibing.

Gem therapists tell of the power of amethysts. In Greek, "amethyst" is "ametusios" and means "remedy against drunkenness." Please don't take this to mean that if you carry an amethyst and you drink, you won't get drunk. It's that carrying an amethyst should give one the strength to refuse a drink and, therefore, prevent intoxication.

‡ WOMEN, TAKE HEED

Women who drink right before menstruating, when their estrogen level is low, get drunk more easily and usually become more nauseated with rougher hangovers than during the rest of their cycle.

‡ EASING THE URGE FOR ALCOHOL

According to medical researcher Carlson Wade, a tangy beverage can ease and erase the urge to imbibe. He recommends a glass of tomato juice with the juice of 1 lemon added and you might also want to throw in a couple of ice cubes. Stir well. Sip as slowly as you would an alcoholic drink.

Glutamine is helpful in easing the urge for alcohol. Take 500 mg three times a day.

‡ Headaches

We said this in our first folk remedy book and it bears repeating. Take a holistic approach to yourself and your headache. Step back and look at the past twenty-four hours of your life. Have you eaten sensibly? Did you get a decent night's sleep? Have you moved your bowels since awakening this morning? Are your sinuses clogged? Do you have a stiff neck? Are there deadlines you need to meet? Do you have added pressures at home or at work? Is there something you're dreading?

Since studies show that more than 90 percent of headaches are brought on by nervous tension, most of our remedies are for the common tension headache and a few for the more serious migraines.

Regularly recurring headaches can be caused by eyestrain, or something as seemingly silly as gum chewing, or a lack of negative ions in the air, or an allergy, or something more serious. We suggest you consult with a health professional to determine the cause of recurring headaches.

Headaches are a headache! Use your instincts, common sense, and patience to find what works best for you.

Research scientists tell us that almonds contain salicylates, the pain-relieving ingredient in aspirin. Eat 15 raw almonds to do the work of 1 aspirin. While it may take a little longer for the headache to vanish, you don't run the risk of side effects. (What the scientists need to find now are fast-acting almonds.)

Get a little bottle of essence of rosemary and rub a small amount of the oil on your forehead and temples, also behind your ears. Then inhale the fumes from the open bottle four times. If your headache doesn't disappear within half an hour, repeat the rubbing and inhaling once more.

This seems to be a favorite of some Indian gurus: In a small pot combine 1 teaspoon of dried basil with 1 cup of hot water, and bring it to a boil. Take it off the stove, then add 2 tablespoons of witch hazel. Let it cool, then saturate a washcloth with the mixture, wring it out, and apply it to the forehead. Bandage it in place and keep it there until the washcloth dries or your headache disappears, whichever comes first.

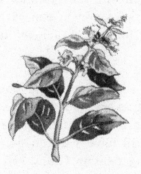

This will either work for you, or it won't. You'll find out quickly and easily. Dunk your hands into water that's as hot as you can stand without scalding yourself. Keep them there for one minute. If you don't start feeling relief within fifteen minutes, go on to another remedy.

If your tension headache seems to stem from the tightness in your neck, use an electric heating pad or a very warm, wet cloth around your neck. The heat should relax you and improve circulation.

If you grow or have fresh mint, take a large mint leaf, bruise it, then roll it up and stick it in your nostril. It is *not* a pretty picture.

A Mexican folk remedy says to paste a fresh mint leaf on the part of the head where the pain is most severe.

In England, the mint leaf is juiced and the juice is used as eardrops to relieve a headache.

Grate a potato (a red one if possible), or an apple, and make a poultice out of it. (See "Preparation Guide.") Apply the poultice to your forehead and bandage it in place, keeping it there for at least an hour.

You might want to try some acupressure to get rid of that headache. Stick out your tongue about ½ inch and bite down on it as hard as you can without hurting yourself. Stay that way for *exactly ten minutes*, not a minute more!

Some people rid themselves of headache pain by taking vitamin C—500 mg every hour—to dilate the constricted blood vessels that are thought to cause the pain. If, after a few hours, you still have a headache, this isn't working for you. Stop taking vitamin C and try another remedy.

The fact that you have this book leads us to believe that you're a person who's interested in and open to all kinds of alternatives, variety, and new adventures. Usually, when a person is adventurous, it extends to his/her eating habits. And so we would like to introduce you to daikon, a Japanese radish (if you aren't already familiar with it). It's delicious eaten raw in salads and wonderful for digestion, especially when eating oily foods.

Meanwhile, back to the headache remedy. Grate a piece of daikon and squeeze out the juice through cheesecloth onto a washcloth. Apply the washcloth to your forehead and bandage in place. It should help draw out the pain.

* * *

While we're talking "exotic edibles," as remedies (see above), you should know about gomasio—that's Japanese for sesame salt. You can buy it at health food stores. The interesting thing about this seasoning is that the oil from the crushed sesame seeds coats the sea salt so that it doesn't cause an excessive attraction for water. In other words, you can season food with it and it won't make you thirsty the way regular salt does.

To get relief from a headache, eat 1 teaspoon of gomasio. Chew it thoroughly before swallowing.

Add ½ teaspoon of angelica (available at health food stores) to ¾ cup of hot water and drink. It not only helps ease the pain of a headache, but it is said to give a person a lighter, happier feeling.

In Jamaica, a popular headache remedy uses the leaf of an aloe vera plant. Carefully cut it in half the long way, and place the gel side on your forehead and temples. Keep it in place with a handkerchief or Ace bandage and let it stay there until your headache is gone.

Niacin has helped many headache sufferers when all else has failed (see "Migraine Headaches"—the first remedy).

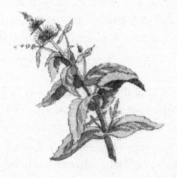

‡ MIGRAINE HEADACHES

Niacin, when taken at the first sign of a migraine, has been known to prevent a full-blown, torturous headache. To prevent or get rid of a headache, take anywhere from 50 to 100 mg at a time. The higher the dosage, the stronger the side effects. For most people, the side effects are felt when they take 100 mg and up. Both of us get the "niacin flush" that makes us look like we've been in the sun too long. It's usually accompanied by itching and/or tingling. It lasts about fifteen minutes and is not at all harmful. Niacinamide is said to be as effective as niacin, but without the side effects. Both are available at vitamin and health food stores.

Bathe your feet in a basin or two plastic shoe boxes filled with very strong, hot, black coffee. Some medical professionals recommend drinking a cup or two of coffee as well. Or, for the same effectiveness, but less caffeine, drink yerba maté, also called Paraguay tea (available at health food stores).

Ready for this one? Sit under a hair dryer. The heat and high-pitched hum may relax the tension that brought on the headache. According to Dr. Robert B. Taylor, our source for this remedy, the dryer brings relief to two-thirds of the migraine sufferers who try it. Your local beauty salon will probably be happy to accommodate you as long as you don't get a headache during their busy time.

NOTE: If you have chemical sensitivities, stay out of a hair salon.

Open a jar of strong mustard and slowly inhale the fumes several times. This has been known to help ease the pain for some people.

Some people have migraines without having severe headaches. Instead, they are troubled by impaired vision—

spots in front of their eyes or seeing double. We heard about a simple remedy. Chew a handful of raisins. Chew them thoroughly before swallowing.

You never know which remedy is going to work best until you try it. Have you tried squatting in 8 inches of hot water (in your bathtub, of course) for twenty minutes?

‡ HEADACHE PREVENTION . . . SORT OF

A three-year study at the University of Michigan showed that students who ate two apples a day had far fewer headaches than those who didn't eat any apples. The apple eaters also had fewer skin problems, arthritic conditions, and colds.

You might want to have an apple for breakfast and one as a late afternoon snack, or one a couple of hours after dinner.

Chances are, eating two apples a day will also prevent constipation, which is a leading cause of headaches.

‡ Heart

‡ HEART ATTACK

If you or someone you're with feels as though they're having a heart attack, call for professional medical help immediately. While you're waiting for help to arrive, squeeze the end of the little finger on the left hand. Squeeze it HARD! Keep squeezing it. This acupressure procedure has been said to save lives.

Like the above remedy, this one has also been known to save lives while waiting for professional help to arrive when someone is having a heart attack. Dr. John R. Christopher, master herbalist, says to put 1 teaspoon of cayenne pepper in a glass of warm water and have the patient force himself to drink it all. Cayenne pepper is hotter than hot and hard to take, but so is having a heart attack.

Or take an aspirin and a magnesium capsule.

‡ HEART HELPERS

According to the results of a study, orchestra conductors live an average of seven and a half years longer than the average person.

To strengthen your heart, tone up your circulatory system, and have some fun, go through the motions of conducting an orchestra. Do it for at least ten minutes a day, or twenty minutes three days a week. Conduct to music that inspires you. If you don't have a baton, use a ruler or a chopstick. Pretend each day of exercise is a command performance. Throw your whole self into it physically and emotionally.

NOTE: If you have a history of heart problems, be sure to check with your doctor before you begin conducting.

Two teaspoons of raw honey a day, either in a glass of water, or straight off the spoon, is thought by many nutritionists to be the best tonic for strengthening the heart, as well as for general physical repair.

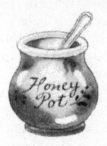

Okay, so you don't want to join a gym. You don't have to. For the best exercise and the perfect body stimulator, just take an old-fashioned walk—make it a brisk old-fashioned walk—daily. *Brisk* means walking a mile every twenty minutes (three miles an hour). It's slower than running or race-walking, and faster than a stroll.

The *New England Journal of Medicine* recently reported the findings of a long-term study of seventy-two thousand women ages forty to sixty-five. The heart attack risk was reduced 30 to 40 percent in the women who did at least three hours of brisk walking a week. The women who walked briskly for five hours or more a week cut heart attack risk by more than 40 percent. In addition to the walking, those who did vigorous exercise for ninety minutes a week cut their risk almost in half. Gardening and housework are considered vigorous exercise. You can have a clean house, a beautiful garden, and a healthy heart.

Incidentally, walking is believed to use the same amount of energy as running.

According to Dr. Richard Passwater, vitamin B_{15} quickens the healing of scar tissue around the heart and also limits the side effects of some heart medications. The suggested dosage is 150 mg a day along with a B-complex vitamin.

This remedy is recommended for people who have a history of heart problems: Right before going to bed, take a ten-minute footbath. Step into calf-high water, as hot as you can take it without scalding yourself. As the minutes pass and the water cools, add more hot water. After ten minutes, step out of the tub and dry your feet thoroughly, preferably with a rough towel. Once your feet are dry, give them a one-minute massage, manipulating the toes as well as the entire foot. This footbath/massage may help circulation, remove congestion around the heart, and pave the way to a peaceful night's sleep.

We recently read a list of supposed benefits of hawthorn berries. We followed up by researching the herb and as a result, we now take hawthorn supplements daily.

Included on that list of benefits were: normalizes blood pressure by regulating heart action; improves heart valve defects; helps people with a lot of stress; strengthens weakened heart muscle, and prevents arteriosclerosis (hardening of the arteries).

Check with your health professional for dosage, depending on your size and the state of your heart health.

‡ ARTERIOSCLEROSIS (HARDENING OF THE ARTERIES)

You might want to check out the remedies in "Heart Helpers," particularly the one above about hawthorn berries. And do something about protecting your arteries against the negative effects of improper diet, lack of exercise, and bad habits (smoking, etc.).

A couple of cloves of garlic a day has been known to unplug arteries. It seems to really do a job cleansing the system, and collecting and casting out toxic waste. Mince the 2 cloves and put them in a half glass of orange juice or water and drink it down. There's no need to chew the pieces of garlic. By just swallowing them, the garlic smell doesn't stay on your breath.

In conjunction with a sensible diet, garlic can also help bring down cholesterol levels in the blood. No wonder this beautiful bulb has a fan club, appropriately called "Lovers of the Stinking Rose."

Rutin is one of the elements of the bioflavonoids. Bioflavonoids are necessary for the proper absorption of vitamin C. Taking 500 mg of rutin daily, with at least the same amount of vitamin C, is said to increase the strength of capillaries, strengthen the artery walls, help prevent hemorrhaging, and help treat arteriosclerosis.

‡ CHOLESTEROL

After researching the subject of cholesterol, our understanding is that there's a harmful cholesterol component (LDL) and a protective cholesterol component (HDL).

Impressive test results build a good case for the effectiveness of lecithin lowering LDL levels and raising HDL levels.

DOSE: 1 to 2 tablespoons of lecithin granules daily, available at health food stores.

The American Journal of Clinical Nutrition mentions that raw carrots not only improve elimination because of their high fiber content, but may also lower cholesterol. Test subjects who ate 2 carrots for breakfast for three weeks reduced their serum cholesterol level by 11 percent.

You may want to scrub the carrots you eat instead of peeling them. The peel is rich in B_1 (thiamine), B_2 (riboflavin), and B_3 (niacin). If you can get organically grown carrots, do so.

It seems that very small amounts of chromium are vital for good health. A deficiency in chromium may be linked to coronary artery disease. Take 1 to 2 tablespoons of brewer's yeast daily (be sure to read labels and select the brewer's yeast with the highest chromium content), or a handful of raw sunflower seeds. The chromium, like the lecithin, is said to lower the LDL cholesterol level and raise the HDL cholesterol level. If you plan on doing this, get your doctor's approval.

Oats can bring down blood cholesterol levels, Dr. Hans Fischer, nutritionist at Rutgers University, concluded after studying results done with test groups. One can reap this benefit by eating oatmeal or any other form of oats two or three times a week.

According to Dr. James W. Anderson, professor of medicine and clinical nutrition at the University of Kentucky College of Medicine, "including a cup of beans in your diet per day helps to stabilize blood sugars and lowers cholesterol." This benefit can be attributed to dry beans, such as pinto, rather than green beans.

This remedy comes from a very recent report. The report falls into the you-can-go-crazy-with-all-of-this category.

Dr. Scott Grundy, professor at the University of Texas Health Science Center in Dallas, says that the new findings show that *mono*unsaturated fatty acid found in olive oil and peanut oil is more effective in reducing artery-clogging cholesterol levels of blood than *poly*unsaturated fats such as corn oil and sunflower oil.

‡ PALPITATIONS

If you have palpitations (and who hasn't at one time or another), take a holistic approach to find the cause. Was it the MSG in the Chinese food you had for lunch? Or the caffeine in the chocolate you pigged out on? Pressure at the office? Cigarette smoke? Sugar? Work at figuring it out so that you learn what not to have next time.

Meanwhile, here's a natural sedative to subdue the thumping. Steep 2 chamomile tea bags in 2 cups of just-boiled water. Steam a few shredded leaves of cabbage. Then, in a soup bowl, combine the steamed leaves with the chamomile tea. This tea-soup may not taste good, but it can help overcome those skipped heartbeats.

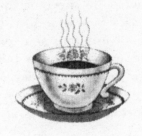

‡ Hemorrhoids

Put the tobacco from 2 cigarettes in a pan, add 4 tea-spoons of butter, and let the mixture simmer for a couple of minutes. Next, pour the hot liquid through a strainer onto a sanitary napkin. When it's cool enough, apply it to the hemorrhoid area. Whip up a fresh batch three times a day.

WARNING: Once you start doing this, you may not want to stop. Well, don't they say tobacco is habit-forming?

A consulting doctor for the Denver Broncos and Denver Nuggets has had success in speeding up athlete's hemorrhoid healing processes with vitamin C baths. The doctor recommends 1 cup of ascorbic acid powder to every 5 quarts of cool bathwater. Sit in the tub for fifteen minutes at a time, two or three times a day. Ascorbic acid powder is expensive. If you can fit your tushy into a basin with ½ cup of the powder and 2½ quarts of cool water, you'll save a fortune.

Take advantage of the healing properties of the enzymes in papaya by drenching a wad of sterilized cotton in pure papaya juice. Position it on the hemorrhoid area and secure it in place. The juice should help stop the bleeding and bring the irritation under control.

How are you at ice carving? Carefully carve or melt an ice cube down to the size and shape of a bullet. Use it as a suppository. The cold may give you a start, but it may also start reducing the swelling and help to heal the hemorrhoids.

‡ Herpes (All Kinds—Genitalis, Simplex, Etc.)

Twenty million Americans (one out of every five sexually active adults) have herpes. Each year three hundred thousand to five hundred thousand more get it.

We spoke with a man who did extensive research and came up with a remedy for overcoming the symptoms (fever blisters, cold sores, etc.) of herpes. He tested it and had friends test it. The results were impressive. But first the remedy, next the explanation, and then more about the results.

Do not eat nuts, chocolate, or (sorry, Mom) chicken soup. At the first sign of a herpes flare-up, eat 1 pound of steamed flounder. That's it. That's the remedy.

The explanation in simple terms, as best as we understand it, is that there's a certain balance in the body between two amino acids—arginine and lysine. To contract herpes and to have the symptoms recur, one's body has to have a high level of arginine compared with the level of lysine. The secret, then, is to reduce the amount of arginine (eliminate nuts, chocolate, and chicken soup) and increase the amount of lysine (eat flounder). The pound of flounder has 11,000 mg of lysine. You can take lysine tablets, but you would have to take so many of them, and besides, they contain binders and other things you just don't need. Also, the tablets are not as digestible or as absorbable as the lysine in flounder. By steaming the fish, you retain of the nutrients. You can add the sauce of your choice to the flounder after it's been steamed.

As for results, the man and his friends have had symptoms disappear overnight after eating flounder and *never* eating nuts, chocolate, and (oh, how we hate to say it) chicken soup.

✠ Hiccups

Locate the area about 2 to 3 inches above your navel and between the two sides of your rib cage. Press in with the fingers of both of your hands and stay that way long enough to say to yourself: one, two, three, four, I don't have the hiccups anymore. If you still have them, try reciting "The Rime of the Ancient Mariner."

Close your eyes, hold your breath, and think of ten bald men. Let us start you off: Sean Connery, Montel Williams, Danny Devito, Paul Shaffer, Ainsley Harriott . . .

Pardon our name-dropping, but . . . When we were on the *Today* show, Jane Pauley told us that her husband, Garry Trudeau, gets painful hiccups. His remedy is to put a teaspoon of salt on half a lemon and then suck the juice out of the lemon.

Our great-aunt Molly used to soak a cube of sugar in fresh lemon juice and then let it dissolve in her mouth. She did it to get rid of the hiccups. She also did it as a shortcut whenever she drank tea.

Just visualizing a rabbit . . . its cute little face, quivering nose, and white whiskers . . . has been known to make the hiccups disappear.

One of the most common remedies for hiccups is a teaspoon of granulated sugar. It supposedly irritates the throat, causing an interruption of the vagus nerve impulse pattern that is responsible for triggering the spasms of the diaphragm. (Just reading the previous sentence aloud may help you get rid of the hiccups.) In Arabia, people have been known to use sand in place of sugar. We haven't tried either remedy since we don't eat sugar and we don't go to the beach.

Another way you might interrupt the diaphragmatic spasms is by holding your arms above your head and panting like a dog. Well, you may not get rid of the hiccups, but you may end up with some table scraps.

Lay a broom on the floor and jump over it six times. If you want to update this remedy, try jumping over a vacuum cleaner. For all you rich people, jump over your maid.

Turn yourself into a "T" by spreading out your arms. Then give a big yawn.

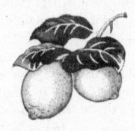

Pretend you're chewing gum while your fingers are in your ears, gently pressing inward. "What? I can't hear you. My fingers are in my ears."

‡ WHEN SOMEONE ELSE HAS THE HICCUPS . . .

Take something cold that's made of metal—a spoon is good—tie a string around it, and lower it down the hiccupper's back.

Suddenly accuse the hiccupper of doing something (s)he did not do. "You left the water running in the tub!" "You borrowed money from me and forgot to pay it back!"

‡ Indigestion

In our great land of plenty, one of the most common ailments is indigestion.

Persistent indigestion may be due to a food allergy. You may need a health professional to help you check it out. Severe indigestion may be something a lot more serious than you think. Seek professional help immediately.

CAUTION: Never take a laxative when you have severe stomach pain.

Mild indigestion usually produces one or a combination of the following symptoms: stomachache, nausea and vomiting, gas and/or heartburn.

Relief may be a page or two away.

When you have stomach cramps caused by indigestion, take 1 teaspoon of apricot brandy as your after-dinner drink.

In the case of acid indigestion, chew dry rolled oats. After thoroughly chewing a teaspoon, swallow them. The oats not only soothe the acid condition, they also neutralize it.

We keep daikon in the refrigerator at all times. It's a Japanese radish . . . white, crisp, delicious, and available at your greengrocer or Asian market. It's an effective digestive aid, especially when eating heavy, deep-fried foods. Either grate 1 to 2 tablespoons or have a couple of slices of the daikon with your meal. It also helps detoxify animal protein and fats.

When you have a white-coated tongue, bad breath, and a headache, it's probably due to an upset stomach. A wise choice of herbs would be sage. Sip a cup of sage tea slowly. (See "Preparation Guide.")

We have come across some strange-sounding remedies for which there seem to be no logical explanation. We've included a few of them, simply because they sometimes work. This is one of them: when your stomach aches, tie a red string around your waist. If the pain disappears, fine. If not, go on to another remedy.

When you have a sour stomach, chew a few anise seeds, cardamom seeds, or caraway seeds. They'll sweeten your stomach and your breath as well.

Like rolled oats (one of the previous remedies), raw potato juice also neutralizes acidity. Grate a potato and squeeze it through cheesecloth to get the juice. Dilute 1 tablespoon of potato juice with ½ cup of warm water. Drink it slowly.

Take a wire hairbrush or a metal comb and brush or comb the backs of your hands for three to four minutes. It's supposed to relieve that sluggish feeling one gets from eating one of those old-fashioned, home-cooked, the-cholesterol-can-kill-ya' meals.

This was recommended to us for a nervous stomach. Add ¼ teaspoon of oregano and ½ teaspoon of marjoram to 1 cup of hot water. Let it steep for ten minutes. Strain and sip slowly. Two hours later, if you still have stomach uneasiness, drink another cup of the mixture.

This remedy from India is recommended for quick relief after a junk-food binge. Crush 1 teaspoon of fenugreek seeds and steep them in 1 cup of just-boiled water for five minutes. Strain and drink slowly. One should feel better in about ten minutes.

According to a Chinese massage therapist, if you are having stomach discomfort, there will be tender areas at the sides of your knees, just below the kneecaps. As you massage those spots and the tenderness decreases, so should the corresponding stomachache.

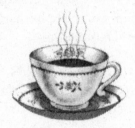

‡ INDIGESTION PREVENTION

A doctor we know practices preventive medicine on himself before eating Szechuan or Mexican food or any other "hot" food that would ordinarily give him an upset stomach. He takes 1 tablespoon of extra-virgin, cold-pressed olive oil about fifteen minutes before the meal.

We've heard that 1 teaspoon of whole white mustard seeds taken before a meal may help prevent stomach distress.

‡ NAUSEA AND VOMITING

When you have an upset stomach and you're feeling nauseated, take a carbonated drink—seltzer, club soda, Perrier, or some ginger ale. If you don't have any of those, and you're not on a sodium-restricted diet, mix 1 teaspoon of baking soda with 1 glass of cold water and drink slowly. Within a few minutes, you should burp and feel better.

Drink 1 cup of yarrow tea (available at health food stores). This herb is known to stop nausea in next to no time. It's also wonderful for helping tone up the digestive system.

When the food you ate seems to be lying on your chest, or you have a bad case of stomach overload and you know you'd feel much better if you threw up, reach for the English mustard. It's available at food specialty shops. Drink 1 teaspoon in a glass of warm water. If you don't upchuck in ten minutes, drink another glass of this mustard water. After another ten minutes, if it still hasn't worked, the third time should be the charm. I'm getting nauseated just thinking about all the watered-down mustard.

To help ease a severe bout of vomiting, warm ½ cup of vinegar, saturate a washcloth in it, and place the moist cloth on your bare stomach with a hot water bottle on top of the cloth.

‡ GAS/FLATULENCE

Are you sure it's gas and not your appendix? To test for appendix problems, in a standing position, lift your right leg and then quickly jut it forward as though kicking something. If you have an excruciating, sharp pain anywhere in the abdominal area, it may be your appendix, in which case, seek medical attention immediately. If there is no sharp pain when you kick, it's probably just gas, but you may want to check with your doctor to be sure.

By now, you probably know which foods give you gas and which meals may prove lethal. But do you know about food combining? The library has lots of books with information on the subject, and there are simple, inexpensive charts sold at health food stores. If you follow proper food combining—for example, wait two hours after eating regular food before eating fruit—you shouldn't ever have a problem with gas. It's not always convenient to stick to good combinations. Here are some remedies for when your food combining is less than perfect and as a result, you're cooking with gas.

When you know you're eating food that's going to make you and everyone around you sorry you ate it, take 2 charcoal tablets or capsules as soon as you finish your meal. It's important to take the charcoal quickly because gas forms in the lower intestine and if you wait too long, the charcoal can't get down there fast enough to help.

WARNING: Do not take charcoal capsules or tablets often. They are powerful adsorbents and will rob you of nutrients you need.

Each one of the following seeds is known to give fast relief from the pain of gas: anise seeds, caraway seeds, dill seeds, and fennel seeds (available at health food stores). To release the essential oils from any of those seeds, gently crush 1 teaspoon and add it to a cup of just-boiled water. Let it steep for ten minutes. Strain and drink. If the gas pains don't disappear right away, drink another cup of the seed tea before eating your next meal.

The unripe berries of a pimento evergreen tree are called allspice. It was given its name because it tastes like a combination of spices: cloves, juniper berries, cinnamon, and pepper. Allspice is said to be effective in treating flatulent indigestion. Add 1 teaspoon of powdered allspice to a cup of just-boiled water and drink. If you have the dried fruit, chew ½ teaspoon, then swallow.

If you feel you have a gas pocket, or trapped gas, lie down on the floor or on a bed and slowly bring your knees up to your chest to the count of ten, then back down. In between this exercise, massage your stomach in a circular motion, with the top half of your fingers, pressing hard to move that gas around and out.

‡ HEARTBURN

Certain foods may not agree with you, causing a condition known as heartburn. My mother used to get heartburn a lot. I remember asking her, "How do you know when you have it?" My mother would answer, "You'll know!" She was right.

When you have heartburn it's best *not* to lie down. The backflow of stomach acid into the esophagus increases when you lie on your right side, so if you have to lie down, stay on your left side.

Keep chewable papaya tablets with you and at the first sign of heartburn, or any kind of indigestion, pop papaya pills in your mouth, chew, and swallow.

A cup of peppermint tea has been known to relieve the discomfort of heartburn. It helps relieve gas, too.

Eat a teaspoon of gomasio (sesame seeds and sea salt, available at health food stores). Chew it thoroughly before swallowing.

This may not be too appetizing, but it works: swallow a teaspoon or two of uncooked oat flakes, after chewing it thoroughly.

The flow of saliva can neutralize the stomach acids that slosh up and cause heartburn. According to Dr. Wylie Dodds at the Medical College of Wisconsin, chewing gum (we suggest sugarless), can increase the production of saliva eight or nine times, and reduce the damage caused by stomach acids.

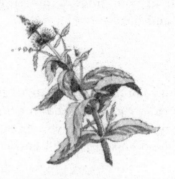

‡ HEARTBURN PREVENTION

Turmeric, a basic ingredient in curries, is also a digestive aid. It stimulates the flow of saliva (saliva neutralizes acid and helps push digestive juices back down where they belong). If you're about to eat food that gives you heartburn, spice up the food with turmeric. If it's not an appropriate ingredient for the food, take 2 or 3 turmeric capsules, available at health food stores, before the meal.

‡ Infants and Children

Every baby-care book tells you to "childproof" your home. Make a crawling tour of each room in your house in order to see things from a child's-eye view. Once you're aware of the danger zones, you can eliminate them by covering wires, nailing down furniture, etc. Do this every four to six months as the child grows, and is able to reach more things.

Still, no matter how childproof a place is, a mishap can happen. We suggest that parents have a first-aid book handy and/or take a first-aid course through the local American Red Cross.

It's also very important to keep a list of the following emergency numbers near every telephone in the house:

- Pediatrician
- Poison Control Center
- Police
- Fire Department
- Hospital
- Pharmacy
- Dentist
- Neighbors (with cars)

In terms of home remedies for common conditions, we caution you that children's systems are much more delicate than ours. While lots of the remedies throughout the book can certainly be applied to youngsters, use good common sense in prescribing doses and strengths. In all cases, check with the pediatrician first.

One major caution: NEVER GIVE HONEY TO A CHILD UNDER ONE YEAR OLD! Spores found in honey have been linked to botulism in babies.

Here are some remedies specifically for children's ailments. They should help you as well as your child to get through those tough times.

‡ ATTENTION DEFICIT AND HYPERACTIVITY DISORDER (ADHD)

If your child has been diagnosed with ADHD, chances are you are looking for an answer so that your child doesn't have to start taking Ritalin, or can be taken off that drug. Have you checked out possible causes like the following: toxic-metal excess, pesticides in the home, behavioral interaction issues in the home and at school, malnutrition, allergies (including those to sweets, milk, and cheese), and gluten intolerance? While your child's diet may play a major part in causing and overcoming this condition, you may not know that several studies point to a connection between children with ADHD and an omega-3 fatty acid deficiency. According to a paper published in *Physiology & Behavior* by a research team from the Department of Foods and Nutrition at Purdue University, boys with lower levels of omega-3 fatty acids in their blood showed more problems with behavior, learning, and health than those with higher total levels of omega-3 fatty acids.

You may want to find out more about this and then consider adding flaxseed oil, the richest source of omega-3 essential fatty acids, to your child's daily diet. For more flaxseed information, see the "Sensational Six" chapter.

‡ APPETITE STIMULANT

Prepare a cup of chamomile tea and add $\frac{1}{16}$ teaspoon of ground ginger. An herbalist recommends 1 teaspoon of the warm tea half an hour before meals to stimulate a child's appetite.

‡ BEDWETTING

This exercise strengthens the muscles that control urination: starting with the first urination of the day, have the child start and stop urinating as many times as possible until (s)he has finished. If you make it into a game, counting the number of starts and stops, the child might look forward to breaking his or her own record each time. It's important, however, not to pressure the child into feeling inadequate if (s)he finds this exercise difficult.

‡ CHICKEN POX

Of course a child with chicken pox should be in bed, kept warm, and on a light diet, including lots of pure fruit juices. Yarrow tea, according to herbalists, seems to be the thing for children's eruptive ailments. Add 1 tablespoon of dried yarrow (available at health food stores) to 2 cups of just-boiled water and let it steep for ten minutes. Strain, then add 1 tablespoon of raw honey. NOTE: NEVER GIVE HONEY TO A CHILD UNDER ONE YEAR OLD. Give the child ½ cupful three or four times a day.

To relieve the itching, a pediatrician recommends a spritz of ordinary spray starch on the itchy areas.

‡ COLDS

According to a study published by two doctors in a respected scientific journal, zinc gluconate lozenges can shorten the duration of a cold dramatically. The lozenges (honey-flavored are the best; lemon are the pits) should not be taken on an empty stomach. Even if the child is not eating much because of the cold, have him or her eat half a fruit before sucking a lozenge.

DOSE: If a child weighs less than 60 pounds, (s)he should take 1 to 3 zinc lozenges—as tolerated—23 mg each, per day—no more. For teenagers, the maximum dose is 3 to 6 lozenges—as tolerated—23 mg each, per day.

IMPORTANT: Do not give the child lozenges for more than two days in a row.

‡ COLIC

A popular European colic calmer is fennel tea. Add ½ teaspoon of fennel seeds to 1 cup of just-boiled water and let it steep for ten minutes. Strain the liquid tea into the baby's bottle. When it's cool enough to drink, give it to the baby. If (s)he's not thrilled with the taste of fennel, try dill seeds instead.

Caraway seeds are said to bring relief to colicky kids (and parents and neighbors). Add 1 tablespoon of bruised caraway seeds to 1 cup of just-boiled water. Let it steep for ten minutes. Strain and put 2 teaspoons of the tea into the baby's bottle. When it's cool enough to drink, give it to the baby.

If you are breast-feeding your baby and (s)he is colicky, try eliminating milk from your diet. There's a 50/50 chance that if you no longer drink milk, the baby will no longer have colic. Be sure, however, to eat calcium-rich foods such as canned salmon, canned sardines, sunflower and sesame seeds, almonds, whole grains, green leafy vegetables, soy products including tofu, and molasses.

Milk isn't the only thing to eliminate from your diet. You should also avoid foods that may be hard for you and your baby to digest: bell (green) peppers, beans, cucumbers, eggs, chocolate, onions, leeks, garlic, eggplant, lentils, zucchini, tomatoes, sugar, coffee, alcoholic beverages—and go easy on the amount of fruit you eat. Remember, it's not forever . . . the diet restrictions *or* the colic!

‡ COUGH

Add ½ teaspoon of anise seeds and ½ teaspoon of thyme to 1 cup of just-boiled water. Let it steep for ten minutes. Stir it, strain, and let cool. Then add a teaspoon of honey.

DOSE: 1 tablespoon every half hour. THIS IS FOR CHILDREN ABOVE THE AGE OF TWO YEARS OLD.

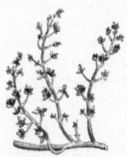

A woman from Oklahoma called to tell us that whenever her child gets a cough that acts up at night, she loosely ties a black cotton thread around the child's neck. IT MUST BE BLACK. This woman said she tried other colors and nothing but the black works.

We were intrigued with the remedy and tested it on our friend's child. It worked like magic. We researched it and found a printed source that credited it to shamans in ancient Egypt.

‡ CROUP

Scottish folk healers treat the croup by wrapping a piece of bacon (uncooked, of course) around the child's neck, bundling him up in a blanket and taking him into a steamy bathroom for a few minutes.

It's something to do till the doctor arrives.

‡ DIARRHEA

From the Pennsylvania Dutch comes this children's remedy for diarrhea. In a warmed cup of milk, add 1/16 teaspoon of cinnamon. The child should drink as much as possible.

Raspberry-leaf tea is excellent for treating diarrhea. Combine 1/2 ounce of dried raspberry leaves with 1 cup of water and simmer in an enamel or glass saucepan for twenty-five minutes. Strain and let the liquid cool to room temperature.

DOSE: For a baby under one year, 1/2 teaspoon four times a day; for a child over one year, 1 teaspoon four times a day.

‡ DIGESTION

If a baby can't seem to keep his food down, you may want to try putting a teaspoon of carob powder in the baby's formula. In some instances it may make the difference.

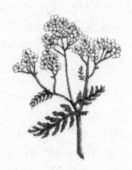

‡ FOREIGN SUBSTANCE IN THE NOSE

Lots of kids stick things up their nose. Lydia put a yankee bean in her nostril when she was three years old, and it began to take root. Luckily, our father noticed that she was sitting still for more than thirty seconds at a time, so he realized something was wrong.

Before you take the child to the doctor to perform a yankee beanectomy, open the child's mouth, place your mouth over it, and briskly blow once. Your gust of breath may dislodge the object from the child's nostril. If it doesn't after that first try, seek medical attention.

‡ MEASLES

Yarrow tea is good for eruptive ailments (see "Chicken Pox" earlier). To strengthen the child's eyes, which are usually affected when one has the measles, and to ease the discomfort in them, make sure the child gets food rich in vitamin A—carrot juice, cantaloupe, and green and yellow fruit.

‡ PAIN AND DISCOMFORT

When baby is teething or has mild colic, or is just irritable because of indigestion or disturbed sleep, steep a chamomile tea bag in a cup of hot water. If the problem is indigestion, throw in a small piece of fresh ginger. After steeping for about ten minutes, take out the tea bag and the ginger. Give the baby a teaspoon of the tea every fifteen minutes until (s)he seems better.

‡ PIMPLY-FACED INFANTS

It's common to see infants with an outbreak of pimples. According to a folk remedy from the 1600s, gently dab the premature case of acne with mother's milk. If you're not nursing the baby, use a few drops of whole milk (not skim milk). Or, gently dab the baby's outbreak with the baby's own wet diaper. The urine has healing antibodies.

‡ PRICKLY HEAT

Gently rub the afflicted area with the red side of a piece of watermelon rind. It should stop the itching and help dry out the rash.

‡ SUNBURN (SEE "BURNS" CHAPTER—SUNBURN PREVENTION/SKIN PROTECTION)

‡ TONSILLITIS

We've been told about lots of cases of swollen tonsils because of an intolerance for milk. That's easy enough to test. Simply eliminate milk from the child's diet and check the results within a day or two. If the child does not assimilate milk properly, there are many other wonderful sources of calcium and it is no big deal for a child not to have milk. Sunflower and sesame seeds are rich in calcium. So are almonds, green leafy vegetables, canned salmon, sardines, molasses, and whole grains. There are also supplements: bonemeal, dolomite, and calcium lactate. Check with a health professional.

Master herbalist Dr. John R. Christopher says that puberty will be easier to go through if the teenagers still have their tonsils. The girls will have easier menstrual periods and the boys will have less chance for prostate malfunction. The reason is that the tonsils are the filtering system for the reproductive organs and are needed by the body.

‡ WARTS

The power of the mind and creative imagery is most effective when it comes to making a child's wart disappear.

Take a piece of tracing or tissue paper, put it on the

child's wart, and with a pencil, trace the wart. Take your child and the paper with the traced-on wart into the bathroom. Then be sure to impress upon the child, "Only Mommy or Daddy can do this." While the child watches, burn the tracing paper and flush away the ashes. In about a week, the wart should be gone.

‡ Kidney and Bladder

Lots of folk remedies include the use of apple cider vinegar to help flush the kidneys and to provide a natural acid. Dosage varies from source to source. We think it makes most sense to take 1 teaspoon of apple cider vinegar for every 50 pounds you weigh, and add it to 6 ounces of water. In other words, if you weigh 150 pounds, the dosage would be 3 teaspoons of vinegar in 6 ounces of water. Drink it twice a day, before breakfast and before dinner. Keep it up for two days, then stop for four days. Continue this two-days-yes/four-days-no cycle as long as you feel you need it.

Aduki (or azuki) beans, found in health food stores, are used in the Orient as food and medicine. They're excellent for treating kidney problems. Rinse a cupful of aduki beans. Combine the cup of beans with 5 cups of water and boil for one hour. Strain the aduki-bean water into a jar. Drink ½ cup of aduki water at least a half hour before meals. Do this for two days—six meals. To prevent the aduki water from spoiling, keep the jar in the refrigerator, then warm the water before drinking.

Our gem therapist friend recommends wearing jade against the skin to help heal kidney and bladder problems. If your mate reads this and surprises you with a piece of jade jewelry, chances are you'll start to feel better immediately.

‡ INCONTINENCE

This remedy comes from the Hottentot tribe of South Africa, where buchu shrubs grow. Steep 1 tablespoon of buchu leaves (available at health food stores) in 1 cup of just-boiled water for half an hour.

DOSE: 3 to 4 tablespoons, three to four times a day. Buchu leaves are known to be helpful for many urinary problems including inflammation of the bladder and painful urination as well as incontinence.

Women, See SEX chapter—For Women Only—"Muscle Strengthener" for bladder control.

‡ BEDWETTING

Just when you may have thought that nothing could help, heeeeeere's uva ursi! This herb is said to strengthen the urinary tract and, taken in small doses, has been known to end bedwetting.

Add 1 tablespoon of the dried uva ursi leaves or 1 tea bag to 1 cup of just-boiled water and steep for five minutes. Strain into a jar.

DOSE: 1 tablespoon before each meal every day for six weeks. (Uva ursi is available at health food stores.)

NOTE: Arbutin, the main component of the herb uva ursi, may cause the urine to turn brownish in color. It's absolutely nothing to worry about.

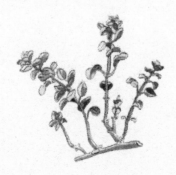

ANOTHER NOTE: We do not list this as a children's bed-wetting remedy because none of our sources mentioned it for children. The herb may be too strong for their delicate systems.

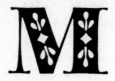

‡ Male Problems

‡ ENLARGED PROSTATE

It is estimated that one out of every three men over the age of sixty has some kind of prostate problem.

We strongly suggest that if you are suffering with pain, burning, testicular or scrotal swelling, or any other prostate-related symptoms, you have your condition evaluated by a health professional.

Grate part of a yellow onion and squeeze it through cheesecloth—enough for a tablespoon of onion juice. Take 1 tablespoon of onion juice twice a day.

In extremely painful cases, get slippery-elm capsules at a health food or vitamin store, take the capsules apart—enough for ½ teaspoon of the slippery-elm powder—and mix the powder with 6 ounces of (preferably distilled) water. Drink the mixture before breakfast and a couple of hours after dinner.

Asparagine, a health-giving alkaloid found in fresh asparagus, is said to be a healing element for prostate conditions. Use a juicer and juice equal amounts of fresh asparagus, carrots, and cucumber—enough for an 8-ounce glass of juice.

Organic vegetables are preferable. If not available, wash

the asparagus thoroughly, scrub the carrots, and peel the cucumber. Drink a glass of the juice daily.

A teaspoon of unrefined sesame oil taken every day for one month has been known to reduce an enlarged prostate back to normal.

A warm milk compress is soothing when applied to the prostate area. Warm, do not boil, one glass of milk. Saturate a white towel in it and when you apply it to the appropriate area, put a hot water bag on top to keep the towel warmer longer.

Lecithin (available at health food stores) comes highly recommended from many sources. Take 1 lecithin capsule—1200 mg each—three times a day, after each meal, or 1 to 2 tablespoons of lecithin granules daily.

‡ PROSTATE CONGESTION

If your doctor hasn't already told you, eliminate all coffee and alcoholic beverages from your diet.

And now for a self-help prostatic massage: lie down on the floor on your back. Put the sole of one foot against the sole of the other foot so that you're at your bowlegged best. While keeping the soles of your feet together, extend your legs as far as possible and then bring them in as close as possible to your chest. Do this "extend and bring in" exercise ten times in the morning and ten times at night.

Dr. Ray C. Wunderlich, Jr., of the Wunderlich Center for Nutritional Medicine in St. Petersburg, Florida, recommends that you empty the gland by having ejaculations at a frequency that you can tolerate. It will improve your urinary stream.

‡ PROSTATE PROBLEM PREVENTION

Eat a handful of shelled, unprocessed, unsalted pumpkin seeds each day. The seeds are rich in zinc, magnesium, phosphorus, iron, calcium, protein, unsaturated fatty acid, and vitamins A and B_1. There are many research results now supporting the benefits of pumpkin seeds for maintaining prostate health. Start now.

‡ BLOODY URINE AFTER JOGGING

Some men pass bloody urine after jogging. It's especially common in men who have scrotal varicocele (varicose veins of the testicles). It's usually due to repeated impact of the empty bladder against the prostate. Some doctors recommend that men not empty their bladders completely right before running.

‡ IMPOTENCE (SEE "SEX.")

‡ PREMATURE EJACULATION (SEE "SEX.")

‡ Memory

"I told my doctor that my memory has gotten terrible lately."

"What did the doctor do about it?"

"He made me pay in advance."

Sure, it's easy to make jokes, but we know how frustrating it is to feel your memory is slipping. A remedy for remembering a familiar name, place, or fact is to simply relax and forget that you can't remember. When you're not thinking about it, it will pop into your mind.

Neither of us believes a good or not-so-good memory is a matter of age. We think we're all victims of data overload.

Scientist and great logician Albert Einstein didn't believe in remembering anything he could look up. While that's not always practical, it is a tension-relieving thought.

Meanwhile, we have some remedies that may help you recreate a wonderful memory.

Yerba maté (pronounced mah-tay) is a form of holly and is the national beverage of Paraguay, where it's grown. One of the many positive effects of the herb, according to South American medical authorities, is that it strengthens one's memory. Drink 1 cup early in the day (available at health food stores).

NOTE: Be aware that yerba maté contains caffeine, although less than coffee or regular tea.

Take 1 teaspoon of apple cider vinegar in a glass of room temperature water before each meal. Not only is it said to be an excellent tonic for the memory, but it also curbs the appetite.

Ah, the healing powers of almonds. Eat 6 raw almonds a day to improve your memory.

Our research led us to a Japanese doctor whose records show that he successfully treated more than five hundred patients who were having memory problems. How? Eyebright, the herb best known for treating eye disorders . . . until now. Add ½ ounce of eyebright and 1 tablespoon of clover honey to 1½ cups of just-boiled water. When it's cool, strain the mixture and put it in a bottle. Drink ¾ cup before lunch and ¾ cup before dinner.

Two mustard seeds, taken as you would take pills, first thing every morning, are said to revive one's memory.

Eat a handful of sunflower seeds daily. These seeds are beneficial in many ways, one being memory improvement.

According to a gem therapist, wearing an amethyst helps strengthen one's memory. You just have to remember to wear the amethyst.

Walking increases oxygen flow to the brain . . . and it's never too late! Researchers experimented on adults between the ages of sixty and seventy-five. The group that walked briskly three days a week, starting with fifteen minutes a day and working their way up to walking forty-five minutes a day, had a 15 percent boost in mental functioning. That 15 percent could mean an end to the frustration of *not* remembering things . . . at any age.

What's the most prevalent color in legal pads? In Post-its? Notice a pattern forming here? According to color therapy research, *yellow* most stimulates the brain. Writing on yellow paper may help you better remember whatever it is you've written.

If you don't think that *color* has an impact on us, think again after you read the following: Alexander Schauss, Ph.D. and director of the American Institute for Bio, Social and Medical Research, recommended that Blackfriars Bridge in London be painted a particular shade of blue, called Ertel Blue, to reduce the incidence of suicides off the bridge, the highest of any bridge on the Thames. The bridge was painted Ertel Blue and the effect was dramatic. No suicides were reported from that point on.

AUTHORS' NOTE: Maybe San Francisco should rethink the Golden Gate Bridge!

‡ Motion Sickness Prevention

Constant jarring of the semicircular canals in the ears causes inner balance problems that produce those awful motion sickness symptoms. To avoid that misery, a doctor at Brigham Young University recommends taking 2 or 3 capsules of powdered ginger half an hour before the expected motion. Or: Stir ½ teaspoon of ginger powder into 8 ounces of warm water and drink it about twenty minutes before you travel.

Here's a we-don't-know-why-it-works-but-it-just-seems-to-work remedy: Tape an umeboshi (a Japanese pickled plum) directly on your navel, right before you board a bus, train, car, plane, or ship, and it should prevent motion sickness. Umeboshi plums are available at health food stores and at Asian markets.

Incidentally, the plums are very rich in calcium and iron. Of course, to reap those benefits, one must *eat* them, rather than tape them on one's tummy.

On any form of transportation, sit near a window so you can look out. Focus on things that are far away, not on nearby objects that move past you quickly.

On a plane, to assure yourself of the smoothest flight possible, select a seat that's over the wheels, not in the tail. There's a lot more movement in the tail end of a plane.

This remedy came to us from Hawaii, Afghanistan, and Switzerland. Take a big brown paper bag and cut off and discard the bag's bottom. Then slit the bag from top to bottom so that it's no longer in the round, but instead a long piece of paper. Wrap the paper around your bare chest and secure it in place. Put your regular clothes on top of it and travel that way. It's supposed to prevent motion sickness.

‡ SEASICKNESS

Marjoram tea is said to help prevent seasickness. Have a cup of the tea before hitting the deck.

Take a teaspoon of gomasio (sesame seeds and sea salt, available at health food stores) and keep chewing it as long as you can before swallowing it. It should help rid you of that queasy feeling

‡ JET LAG PREVENTION

Marco Polo, Ferdinand Magellan, and Christopher Columbus—all world travelers, but none of them had to worry about jet lag.

There's no question about it, we are the "jet lag generation." As a result, our remedies don't go back all that far. As with all of our remedies, try the one(s) that make the most sense to you, taking into consideration your own system and how it reacts to things.

This is the U.S. Department of Energy's Anti–Jet Lag Diet to help travelers quickly adjust their bodies' internal clocks to new time zones.

Start three days before departure day. Day 1: Have a high-protein breakfast and lunch, and a high-carbohydrate (no meat) dinner. No coffee except between 3 and 5 P.M.

Day 2: Have very light meals—salads, light soups, fruit, and juices. Coffee only between 3 and 5 P.M.

Day 3: Same as Day 1.

Day 4, departure: (listen up, this gets complex) If you must have a caffeinated beverage, you can have a cup in the morning when traveling west, or between 6 and 11 P.M. when traveling east. Have fruit or juice until your first meal. To know when to have your first meal, figure out when breakfast time will be at your destination. If your flight is long enough, sleep until normal breakfast time at your destination, *but no later* (that's important). Wake up and eat a big, high-protein breakfast. Stay awake and active. Continue the day's meals according to mealtimes at your destination, and you'll be in sync when you arrive. NO ALCOHOL ON THE PLANE!

This is a modified version of the remedy above that may also help minimize jet lag.

As soon as you board the plane, pretend it's whatever time it actually is at your destination. In other words, if you board the plane at 7 P.M. in New York, and you're headed for London where it's 1 A.M., pull down your window shade or wear dark glasses, and, if possible, go to sleep. If you board a plane late that night and it's daylight at your destination, force yourself to stay awake during the flight. Making believe you're in the new time zone at the very start of your trip should help you acclimate quickly.

*   *   *

William F. Buckley got this remedy from a world traveler friend of a British doctor specializing in jet lag.

The theory behind the remedy is that jet lag comes from internal perspiring, which causes a salt deficiency. According to Buckley, the doctor said to put a heaping teaspoon of salt in a cup of coffee the minute you get into the plane, and drink it. Five hours later, drink another cup and you will experience a miracle. The salted coffee will taste like ambrosia. That is your body talking, telling you how grateful it is that you have given it the salt it so badly needs.

NOTE: This is definitely not for anyone who is watching his or her sodium and/or caffeine intake.

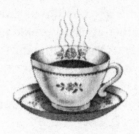

‡ Neck Problems

‡ PAIN-IN-THE-NECK PREVENTION

It's quite common for those of us who are under pressure to have a pain in the neck. People tend to tense up in that area, which is the worst thing to do to yourself. Your neck connects your brain and nervous system to your body. When you create tension in your neck, you impair the flow of energy throughout your system. To prevent tension buildup, do neck rolls. Start with your chin on your chest and slowly rotate your head so that your right ear reaches for your right shoulder, then head back, left ear to left shoulder, and back with your chin on your chest. Do these rolls, slowly, six times in one direction and six times in the opposite direction, morning and evening. You may hear lots of crackling, crunching, and gravelly noises coming from your neck. As tension is released, the noises will quiet. See the next remedy to help rid yourself of gravel.

‡ NECK GRAVEL

If, when you roll your neck around or just turn from side to side, you hear and feel that there's gravel in your neck, do the exercise described above, and eat 3 to 4 cloves of raw garlic a day. You may have to work your way up to that amount. (See "Sensational Six Superfoods"—Garlic, for the easiest way to take raw garlic cloves.)

‡ STIFF NECK

Medicine men from several Native American tribes prescribe daily neck rubs with fresh lemon juice, as well as drinking the juice of half a lemon first thing in the morning and last thing at night.

According to the ancient principles of reflexology, the base of the big toe affects the neck. Rub your hands together vigorously until you feel heat. Now you're ready to massage your big toes with circular motions. Spend a few minutes massaging the bottom of your feet at the base of the toes and the area surrounding them. As a change of pace, you might want to massage the base of your thumbs, also for a few minutes at a time. Keep at it, at least two times a day, every day.

‡ WHIPLASH

Whiplash is the result of neck muscles that were too tense to absorb a sudden thrust. We've been told by medical professionals that a neck collar is the worst thing you can use for whiplash. It doesn't help realign the neck and it doesn't let the body help realign itself. A naturopath, chiropractor, or osteopath can realign the neck vertebrae. During this uncomfortable time, wear a silk scarf. It has been known to help blood circulation and relieve muscle pain and tension in the neck.

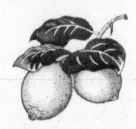

‡ Nervous Tension, Anxiety, and Stress

Sweaty palms, indigestion, hyperventilating, a stiff neck, an ulcer, a dry mouth, a tic—yes, even a canker sore—can be caused by nervous tension, anxiety, and stress.

There are as many symptoms and outward manifestations of anxiety as there are reasons for it. Throughout this book, we address ourselves to the problem at hand, like sweaty palms. In this chapter, we address the problem that may have caused the symptom: nervous tension and stress.

Dr. Joyce Brothers unwinds by doing heavy gardening on her farm. Sailing is a great release for Walter Cronkite. Lawyer F. Lee Bailey pilots his own plane for relaxation.

While not all of us have a plane, a sailboat, or a farm, most of us have a kitchen, a neighborhood health food store, and the following tension-relieving remedies:

A good first step would be to get off products with caffeine. Substitute herbal teas for regular tea and coffee. If you're a chocoholic, check out carob bars when you get a craving for chocolate. Health food stores have a big selection of carob treats that contain no caffeine. The taste and texture of some carob brands are similar to chocolate.

Harried housewives, *do not* paint your kitchens yellow to cheer you up. According to color therapist Carlton Wagner, a yellow room contributes to stress and adds to feelings of anxiety.

Here's a little acupressure to relieve life's pressure. For at least five minutes a day, massage the webbed area between your thumb and index finger of your left hand. Really get in there and knead it. It may hurt. That's all the more reason to keep at it. Gradually, the pain will decrease, so will the tenseness and tightness in your chest and shoulders. Eventually, you should have no pain at all and you should notice a difference in your general relaxed state of well-being.

For a burst of energy without the tension that's usually attached to it, add ⅛ teaspoon of cayenne pepper to a cup of warm water, and drink it down. It's strong stuff and may take a while to get used to, but cayenne is so beneficial, it's worth it. Once you get used to it, increase the amount to ¼ teaspoon, then to ½ teaspoon.

Make two poultices out of a large, raw, grated onion. (See "Preparation Guide.") Place one poultice on each of your calves and leave them there for half an hour. We know, it's hard to believe that onions on your legs can eliminate nervous anxiety, but don't knock it until you try it.

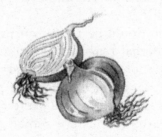

If all of your tension is preventing you from falling asleep, try the tranquilizing effect of a hop pillow. (See "Sleep" for details.)

Let's talk about something lots of you already know about—Valium. Did you know that breast enlargement has been reported in men due to taking Valium? Unfortunately, that's not one of the side effects for women. Oh, but there are some side effects for women. And, there is an alternative that is said to have no side effects. It's called valerian root, the natural forerunner to Valium. Capsules and tablets are available at health food stores. Follow the dosage on the label. Cut and powdered valerian root is available, but the smell is so vile, we can't imagine anyone wanting to make their own tea with it.

Did you know there's a Center for the Interaction of Animals and Society? Well, there is and it's at the University of Pennsylvania, where results of a study showed that looking at fish in a home aquarium is as beneficial as biofeedback and meditation, in terms of relaxation techniques. Yup, just sitting in front of a medium-size fish tank, watching ordinary, nonexotic little fish, relaxed people to the point of considerably improving their blood pressure.

Get a few guppies and pull up a chair! Or, if you have a VCR, there are tapes of fish in aquariums and in the ocean.

Chia seeds are a calmative. Drink a cup of chia-seed tea before each meal. Also sprinkle the seeds on salads.

Alternate-nostril breathing is a well-known yoga technique used to put people in a relaxed state with a feeling of inner peace.

Pay attention; it sounds more complex than it is. Place your right thumb against your right nostril. Place your right ring finger and right pinky against your left nostril. (This is not an exercise for anyone with a stuffed nose.) Inhale and slowly exhale through both nostrils. Now press your right nostril closed and slowly inhale deeply through your left nostril to the count of five. While your right nostril is still closed, press your left nostril closed. With the air in your lungs, count to five. Open your right nostril and exhale to the count of five. Inhale through your right nostril to the count of five. Close both nostrils and count to five. Exhale through the left nostril to the count of five. Keep repeating this pattern for—you guessed it—five minutes. Do it in the morning when you start your day and at day's end.

Kombu is a seaweed. Kombu tea can be a potent nerve tonic. Add a 3-inch strip of kombu to a quart of water and boil it for ten minutes. Drink ½ cup at a time throughout the day. Kombu is available at health food stores and Asian markets.

Do you still have some clothespins hanging around? Take a handful of them and clip them to the tips of your fingers, at the start of your nails of your left hand. Keep them there for seven minutes. Then put those clothespins on the fingers of your right hand for another seven minutes. Pressure exerted on nerve endings is known to relax the entire nervous system.

Do this clothespin bit first thing in the morning, and before, during, or right after a particularly tense situation.

Here's a visualization exercise used by hypnotherapists and at many self-help seminars. Make sure you're not going to be disturbed by telephones, pagers, cell phones, doorbells, dogs, whistling teapots, etc. Sit in a comfortable chair. Close your eyes. Wait! Read this first, then close your eyes. Once your eyes are closed, put all your awareness in your toes. Feel as though nothing else exists but your toes. Completely relax the muscles in your toes. Slowly move up from your toes to your feet, ankles, calves, knees, thighs, genital area, hips, back, stomach, chest, shoulders, arms, hands, neck, jaw, mouth, cheeks, ears, eyes, and brow. Yes, even relax the muscles of your scalp. Now that you're totally relaxed, take three slow, deep breaths, then slowly open your eyes. Now, you go, girl! . . . or guy!

‡ STAGE FRIGHT

Most of us get nervous when we have to do any kind of public speaking. In fact, lots of professional performers get a bad case of butterflies before the curtain goes up.

Here are a couple exercises that can make nervousness a thing of the past.

Before "showtime," stand squarely in front of an immovable wall. Put both your palms on the wall, elbows bent slightly, have your right foot a step in front of the left one, also both legs slightly bent at the knees, and PUSH! PUSH! PUSH! the wall. This flexing of your diaphragm somehow dispels the butterflies.

Remind me to tell you about the time my sister thought a TV studio wall was immovable and it turned out to be part of a set that was quite movable. (That's one show to which we probably won't be invited back.)

A minute before "You're on!" slowly take a deep breath. When no more air will fit into your lungs, hold it for two seconds, then let the air out *very fast*, in one big "whoosh." Do this two times in a row, and you should be ready to go out there in complete control.

‡ Neuralgia

The average human body has forty-five miles of nerves. Neuralgia is an inflammation of a nerve and seems to be caused by poor circulation—too much or too little blood in an area.

To ease the pain of a neuralgia attack, hard-boil an egg. Take off the shell, cut the egg in half, and when it cools enough not to burn you, apply both halves to the trouble spot. By the time the egg cools completely, the pain should be gone.

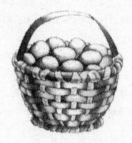

If you have neuralgic pains in the face, let the hot streams of a shower beat against the problem area. Or, you might want to try a hot water compress if you feel that the shower is too much for you to take.

‡ Nosebleeds

When you have a nosebleed, sit or stand. Do not lie down. Do not put your head back. It will cause you to swallow blood.

NOTE: Nasal hemorrhaging—blood flowing from both nostrils—requires immediate medical attention. Rush to the nearest doctor or hospital emergency room.

Also, recurrent nosebleeds may be a symptom of an underlying ailment. Seek appropriate medical attention.

For the *occasional* nosebleed, first thing to do is to gently blow your nose. It will help rid your nostrils of blood clots that may prevent a blood vessel from sealing. Then try any of the following remedies:

In our first book, we reported that a small piece of brown paper from a brown paper bag, placed between the upper lip and the gum, has been known to stop a bloody nose in no time. We have since heard that a dime under the upper lip also stops the nosebleed. If you're outdoors without a paper bag or a dime, a stiff green leaf from a tree can serve the purpose. Place the leaf under your upper lip and press down on it with your finger.

This is a remedy that came to us from the Caribbean islands: Take the pinky finger of the hand opposite the bleeding nostril and tightly tie a string under the pinky's fingernail.

We know that cayenne pepper stops the bleeding of a cut or gash. We've been told that drinking ⅛ teaspoon of cayenne in a glass of warm water will stop a nosebleed.

‡ ‡ ‡

Gem therapists say that a nosebleed can be stopped by placing a piece of pure amber on the nose.

If you happen to get a bloody nose right before making chicken soup, take a piece of the fresh raw chicken and insert it up the bleeding nostril. What we would like to know is, how in the world someone ever discovered this to be an effective remedy for a nosebleed. If you know, please let us know.

Vinegar is said to be very helpful in getting a bloody nose under control. Pour some vinegar on a cloth and wash the neck, nose, and temples with it. Also, mix 2 teaspoons half a glass of warm water and drink it.

‡ PREVENTING NOSEBLEEDS

Bioflavonoids help prevent nosebleeds. Eat at least one citrus fruit a day and be sure to include the white rubbery skin under the peel. It's called the "pith" and it's extremely rich in bioflavonoids. In addition, take a vitamin C supplement with bioflavonoids. Also, add green leafy vegetables—lots of 'em—to your diet. They're rich in vitamin K, needed for the production of prothrombin, which is necessary for blood clotting.

‡ Phlebitis

If you know you have phlebitis, chances are you are under a doctor's care and should be.

After the acute care has been medically completed, pay strict attention to optimal diet, optimal bowel function, optimal weight and exercise, and meticulous body hygiene—nose, ears, mouth, tongue and gums, fingernails, legs, feet, toes, toenails, scrotum or vulva—to prevent complications and recurrence.

Excellent herbs to assist vein health are butcher's broom, hawthorn, and horse chestnut, all available at health food stores. Follow the recommended dosage on the label.

Check with your doctor about the following suggestions. We're certain (s)he will agree that these cannot harm you. And they sure as heck can help dissolve blood clots!

Apply a comfrey poultice on the outside of the affected area. (See "Preparation Guide.")

You should be on a raw vegetable diet. It's important to have leafy greens, plus lots more roughage.

Also, drink lots of fresh juices.

Take 1 tablespoon of lecithin every day.

And surely your doctor told you to elevate the affected area as many hours a day as possible.

‡ Ringworm

A woman called us to share her ringworm remedy: Mix blue fountain pen ink with cigar ashes and put the mixture on the fungus-infected area. The woman said she has never seen it fail. Within a few days the ringworm completely disappears.

If this remedy is going to get you into the habit of smoking cigars, stick with the ringworm, or try the next remedy.

Mince or grate garlic and mix it with an equal amount of petroleum jelly. Apply the mixture to the trouble spots and cover with gauze. Leave it that way overnight. Throughout the day, puncture garlic pearls and rub the oil on the afflicted areas. The garlic should stop the itching and help heal the rash.

‡ Sciatica

Sciatica is a painful condition affecting the sciatic nerve, which is the longest nerve in the body. It extends from the lower spine through the pelvis, thighs, down into the legs, and ends at the heels. We all have some nerve!

Polish folk healers tell their patients who suffer from sciatica to wear long woolen underwear, red only, and carry a raw beet in their hip pocket.

We heard about a man who went from doctor to doctor for help. Nothing worked. As a last resort, the man followed the advice of a folk medicine practitioner who recommended garlic milk. The man minced 2 cloves of garlic, put them in ½ cup of milk, and drank it down (without chewing the pieces of garlic). He had the garlic milk each morning and each evening. Within a few days, he felt some relief. Within two weeks, all the pain had completely disappeared.

Water has tremendous therapeutic value for a sciatic condition. It can reduce the pain and improve circulation. Take a long, hot bath or shower and follow it with a short cold shower. If you can't stand the thought of a cold shower, then follow up the hot bath with ice-cold compresses on the painful areas.

‡ Sex

While we did have "Impotence" under "Male Problems" and "Frigidity" under "Female Problems" in our first folk remedy book, we did not include the subject of "Sex."

During appearances on dozens of radio and television shows, we were constantly asked sex-related questions. As a result, in this book we decided to give the people what they want—more sex! That is, remedies for sexual dysfunctions and some fuel to help rev up the sex drive.

Researchers tell us that about 90 percent of the cases of decreased sexual ability are psychologically caused. Since a psychological placebo has been known to evoke a prizewinning performance, we're including rituals, recipes, potions, lotions, charms, and all kinds of passion-promoting spells.

For history buffs and for history in the buff, we culled the ancient Greek, Egyptian, Indian, and Asian sex secrets that are still being used today.

So, if you did but don't; should but won't; can't but want to; or do but don't enjoy it, please read on. Help and newfound fun may be waiting on the following pages.

‡ FOR MEN ONLY

‡ Impotence: Organic or Psychological?—A Test

Most men have about five erections every night in their sleep. No matter how uptight they might be, and no matter what trouble they might be having with erections while awake, men who suffer from psychological impotency will have firm erections every night in their sleep.

To test for these erections, get a roll of postage stamps (any denomination) and wrap it in a single thickness around the shaft of the penis. Tear off the excess stamps, then tape the two ends (the first and the last stamps) around the penis, firmly but not too tight. Pleasant dreams!

When a nighttime erection occurs, the increased diameter of the penis should break the stamps along the line of one of the perforations. If impotency is organically caused, you will not have nightly erections and the stamps will be intact in the morning.

The "stamp act" should be repeated every night for two to three weeks. If, each morning, the stamps are broken along a perforation, chances are you have a normal capability for erections, and impotency is psychologically caused. Sometimes just knowing that everything is working well organically will give you the confidence and assurance you need to help you rise to the occasion.

‡ The Fear of Failure

In the Mexican pharmacopoeia, damiana is classified as an aphrodisiac and a tonic for the nervous system. It's been known to be an effective remedy for "performance anxiety."

Add a teaspoon of damiana leaves (available at health food stores) to a cup of just-boiled water. Let it steep for ten minutes. Strain and drink before breakfast, on a daily basis.

‡ Amazonico Impotence Remedy

El Indio Amazonico, a Bogotá *botánico* (medicine man), advises his impotent patients to not even try to have sex for thirty days. During that time, he suggests they eat goat meat every day, in addition to bulls' testicles ("mountain oysters"). He also recommends drinking tea made of cinnamon sticks and cups of cocoa. When the abstention period is over, El Indio instructs his patients to rub a small amount of petroleum jelly mixed with a bit of lemon juice around— but not on—the scrotum. Then they're on their own.

‡ Love Longer

Eat a handful of raw, hulled pumpkin seeds every day. (The cooking process may destroy some of the special values of the seeds, so steer clear of the roasted ones.) Pumpkin seeds contain large amounts of zinc, magnesium, iron, phosphorus, calcium, vitamin A, and the B vitamins. According to a German medical researcher, there are one or more substances not yet isolated that have vitalizing and regenerative effects and actually cause additional sex hormones to be produced. Many health authorities agree that a handful of pumpkin seeds a day may help prevent prostate problems and impotence. Pass the pumpkin seeds!

‡ Voice and Vitality

It is said that the higher a man's voice, the lower his masculine vitality. The theory is based on the fact that the vortex at the base of the neck and the vortex in the sex center are directly connected and affected by each other. Men, lower your voice and you'll increase the speed of vibration in these vortexes, which, in turn, may increase your sexual energy.

‡ Recipe for Sexual Stamina

Hindi records, circa tenth century, tell about men who went to view the famous Temple of Khajuraho in India to study its pornographic stone carvings depicting every known position of love. In order to have the stamina to test the positions, they were fed this eggplant dish:

Slice an eggplant and cover with butter and minced chives on both sides. Brown the slices and cover with a spicy curry sauce.

The recipe (unspecific as it is) has been passed down from generation to generation, along with its reputation for making old men young again.

‡ *Stay out of Hot Water*

Fast cold showers do not cool or dampen one's sexual desire. *Au contraire!* Short applications of cold water, particularly on the nape of the neck, are sexually stimulating.

‡ *Stronger Erection*

Most men get a stronger erection and feel more of a sensation when their bladder is full. However, some positions may be uncomfortable if it's very full.

NOTE: Men with prostate problems should not practice this technique.

‡ *Premature Ejaculation*

According to sex therapists, premature ejaculation seems to be one of the easiest conditions to cure, simply by behavior modification. This is Masters and Johnson's conditioning treatment: Enlist the assistance of your mate, who should be very willing to comply. Lie on your back with your legs straddling your partner. Have her stimulate your penis until you feel that orgasm is just around the corner. At that second, give her a prearranged signal. In response to the signal, she should stop stimulating and start squeezing the penis just below the tip. She should squeeze it firmly enough to cause you to lose your erection, but not to cause you pain. When the feeling that you are about to ejaculate leaves you, have her stimulate you again. As before, signal her when orgasm is imminent and, once again, she should stop stimulating and start squeezing the penis. The erection should go down and you will not ejaculate. Keep this up (and down) for a while and soon you will be able to control ejaculation.

The next step is intercourse. As soon as you feel you are about to climax, signal your partner, withdraw from her, and have her squeeze your penis until you lose the erection. Practice makes perfect. Masters and Johnson have reported that in just two weeks of using this behavior modification program, 98 percent of men with premature ejaculation are cured.

‡ The Heart and the Heat of Passion

It's a myth that sex is dangerous to the heart, according to Dr. Richard A. Stein, director of the heart exercise laboratory at the State University of New York Downstate Medical Center.

The stress to the heart is really very mild. The average heart rate increases up to 115 to 120 beats per minute during intercourse—a muscle workload equal to walking up two flights of stairs.

WARNING: If a man is cheating on his mate, the heart rate and risk rises with the excitement and the danger of being caught.

‡ FOR WOMEN ONLY

‡ Overcome Frigidity

In Roman mythology, Anaxarete was so cold to her suitors . . . How cold was she? She was so cold that Aphrodite, the Goddess of Love, turned her into a marble statue. That's cold!

Here is an antifreeze that might work even for Anaxarete: Boil 1 cup of finely minced chive leaves and roots (available at a greengrocer) with 2 cups of champagne. Then simmer until reduced to a thick cupful. Drink it unstrained. It's no wonder this syrup may work. Centuries later, we learned it's rich in vitamin E (the love vitamin). Also, Champagne has always been known to provoke passion. Casanova used it continually in his erotic cookery.

‡ Heighten a Man's Orgasm

Touching a man's testicles before his orgasm is a wonderful way for a woman to greatly excite her lover. It also may hasten as well as heighten the orgasm.

NOTE: Touching the testicles just after orgasm is a no-no. It gives an unpleasant, almost painful sensation.

‡ *Love Elixir for Sexual Responsiveness*

Ancient Teuton brides drank honey-beer for thirty days after their wedding ceremony. It was said to make the bride more sexually responsive. The custom of honey-beer for a month, poetically referred to as a "moon," is the way we got the term "honeymoon."

Rather than go through the big bother of preparing honey-beer the way they did way back when, herbalists simplified it to a tea made from hops and honey.

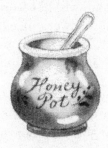

Place 1 ounce of hops (available at health food stores) in a porcelain or Pyrex container. Pour 1 pint of boiling water over the hops, cover, and allow to stand for fifteen minutes, then strain. Add a teaspoon of raw honey to a wineglass of the tea and drink it an hour before each meal. If you prefer warm hops and honey, heat the tea before drinking.

Honey has aspartic acid and vitamin E. Honey and hops contain traces of hormones. All these ingredients are said to stimulate female sexuality. I'll drink to that!

‡ *It Makes Scents*

Have your favorite fragrance linger in the air and help

set the mood for romance. Lightly spray your perfume on a lightbulb—one you plan to leave on. In cold weather, spray your radiator, too.

‡ Fertili-Tea

Add 1 teaspoon of sarsaparilla to 1 cup of just-boiled water and let it steep for five minutes. Strain and drink 2 cups a day.

While sarsaparilla tea may be helpful to a woman who wants to conceive, it should not be given to a man who wants to be potent. Sarsaparilla (available at health food stores) seems to inhibit the formation of sperm.

‡ Fertility Charm

Hundreds of years ago, witches wore necklaces of acorns to symbolize the fertile powers of nature. In some circles it is still believed that by carrying an acorn you will promote sexual relations and conception.

‡ Muscle Strengthener

The ancient Japanese, masters of sensuality, invented Ben Wa Balls. Later, eighteenth-century French women referred to them as *pommes d'amour* ("love apples"). Doctors throughout the world have recommended them for their therapeutic value.

When these brass (or sometimes gold-plated steel) balls are placed in the vagina, they create a stimulating sensation upon the vaginal wall muscles. To keep them from falling out, the vaginal muscle has to be contracted. This exercise strengthens the muscle, supposedly giving the woman more control over her orgasms.

A strong vaginal muscle is beneficial to pregnant women. They have more control over their bladder, and it's said to make the birth process a little easier. A strong vaginal muscle also helps prevent incontinence.

‡ FOR MEN AND WOMEN

‡ Time for Love

Testosterone, the sexual desire–stimulating hormone, is at its lowest level in the body at bedtime, 11 P.M. It's at its highest level at sunrise. No wonder you may not want to make love during *The Tonight Show*. Instead, try getting up with the roosters, and maybe you and your mate will have something to crow about.

‡ Tea for Two

Turkish women believe fenugreek tea makes them more attractive to men. Besides the sexual energy it may give them, the tea has a way of cleansing the system, sweetening the breath, and helping eliminate perspiration odors.

Men suffering from lack of desire and/or inability to perform have turned to fenugreek tea with success.

Many men with sexual problems lack vitamin A. Fenugreek contains an oil that's rich in vitamin A. Trimethylamine, another substance found in fenugreek, and currently being tested on men, acts as a sex hormone in frogs. If you want to do your own testing, add 2 teaspoons of fenugreek seeds to a cup of just-boiled water. Let it steep for five minutes, stir, strain, add honey and lemon to taste. Drink a cup a day and don't be surprised if you get the urge to make love on a lily pad.

‡ Sexy Clam Bake

Bake the meat of a dozen clams for about two hours at 400 degrees. When the clam meat is dark and hard, take out of oven, let cool, and pulverize it to a powder, either in a blender or with a mortar and pestle. Take ½ teaspoon of the clam powder with water, two hours before bedtime, for one week. This Japanese folk remedy is supposed to restore sexual vitality.

‡ Aphrodisiacs

We heard about a married couple whose idea of "sexual compatibility" is for both of them to get a headache at the same time.

They're the ones who asked us to include aphrodisiacs. The word itself means "any form of sexual stimulation." It was derived from the name Aphrodite, the Goddess of Love, who earned her title by having one husband and five lovers including that handsome Greek guy Adonis. Enough about her!

Here are recipes for you and your mate that can add new vigor and uninhibited sensuality to your love life.

‡ Sensation Stirrer

To get in the mood, get in a warm bath to which you've added 2 drops of jasmine oil, 2 drops of ylang-ylang oil, and 8 drops of sandalwood oil. These essential oils are natural, organic substances that work in harmony with the natural forces of the body. Health food stores carry these "oils of olé!" You might want to save water by bathing together.

‡ The Curse That Renews Sexual Bliss

Ancient mystics used "curses" as a positive way to reverse the negative flow of physical manifestations. In other words, if you're not hot to trot, Curses! The secret of success lies in the emotional charge behind the incantation as you repeat it morning, noon, and right before bedtime:

Eros and Psyche, Cupid and Venus, restore to me
  passion and vitality.
Mars and Jupiter, Ares and Zeus, instill in me strength
  and force.
Lusty waters and penetrating winds, renew my vigor,
  my capacity, my joy.
Cursed be weakness, cursed be shyness,
Cursed be impotence, cursed be frigidity,
Cursed be all that parts me and thee!

‡ Passion Fruit

Fruits beginning with the letter "p" are said to be especially good for increasing potency in men and enhancing sexual energy in women. The fruits we recommend are: peaches, plums, pears, pineapple, papayas, persimmons, and don't forget bananas—uh, pananas.

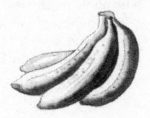

‡ Potion and Chant for Enduring Love

Stir a pinch of ground coriander seeds into a glass of fine red wine while repeating this chant together:
Warm and caring heart
Let us never be apart.
Both sip the wine from the same glass, taking turns. When the wine is all gone, your love should be here to stay.

‡ Native American Passion Promoter

Add 2 tablespoons of unrefined oatmeal and ½ cup of raisins to 1 quart of water and bring it to a boil. Reduce heat, cover tightly, and simmer slowly for forty-five minutes. Remove from heat and strain. Add the juice of 2 lemons and stir in honey to taste. Refrigerate the mixture. Drink 2 cups a day—one before breakfast and another an hour before bedtime.

Oatmeal is rich in vitamin E. Is that where "sow wild oats" comes from?

‡ A Gem of a Gem

According to a gem therapist, wearing turquoise is said to increase its owner's sexual drive.

‡ *The Honeymoon Picker-Upper*

This is an updated recipe of an ancient Druid formula. Sex therapists who prescribe it believe that taking it on a regular basis can generate a hearty sexual appetite.

Mix the following ingredients in a blender for several seconds: 2 level tablespoons of skim milk powder and water according to the skim milk instructions, ¼ teaspoon of powdered ginger, ⅛ teaspoon of powdered cinnamon, 2 tablespoons of raw honey, and a dash of lemon juice, plus any fresh fruit or pure fruit juice you care to add. It's a great snack before the games begin.

‡ Skin

Skin is the largest organ of the body. The average adult has 17 square feet of skin. Thick- or thin-skinned, it weighs about 5 pounds.

Five pounds of skin covering 17 square feet of body surface ... that's a lot of room for eruptions, rashes, scrapes, scratches, splinters, wrinkles, sores, and enlarged pores.

Gimme some skin and we'll give you some remedies!

‡ ACNE

The following acne remedies may not produce dramatic results overnight. Select one and stay with it for at least two weeks. If there's no improvement by then, go on to another remedy.

This South American remedy was given to us by noted herbalist Angela Harris, who has used it to clear up the faces of many a teenager. Wash with mild soap and hot water. Then apply a thin layer of extra-virgin, cold-pressed olive oil. Do not wash it off. Let the skin completely absorb the olive oil. (Angela emphasized the importance of using "extra-virgin olive oil.") Do this three times a day. Angela's experience has been that the skin clears up within a week. For maintenance, wash and oil once a day.

Once a day, take ⅓ cup uncooked oats and, in a blender, pulverize them into a powder. Then add water—a little less than ⅓ cup—so that it becomes the consistency of paste. Apply the paste to the pimples. Leave this soothing and healing mush on until it dries up and starts crumbling off. Wash it all off with tepid water.

NOTE: Always wash your face with tepid water. Hot water can cause the breaking of capillaries, as can cold water.

Using a juice extractor, juice 1 cucumber. With a pastry brush, apply the cucumber juice to the trouble spots. Leave it on for at least fifteen minutes, then wash off with tepid water. Do this daily.

Once a day, boil ⅓ cup of buttermilk. While it's hot, add enough honey to give it a thick, creamy consistency. With a pastry brush, brush the cooled mixture on the acned area. Leave it on for at least fifteen minutes. Wash off with tepid water.

This is an industrial-strength acne remedy taken internally. Before breakfast, or as your breakfast, on the first day, start with 2 teaspoons of brewer's yeast, 1 tablespoon of lecithin granules, and 1 tablespoon of cold-pressed safflower oil, all in one glass of pure apple juice. On the second day, add another teaspoon of brewer's yeast and another teaspoon of lecithin granules. Each day, add another teaspoon of brewer's yeast and lecithin granules until you're taking 2 tablespoons (6 teaspoons) of brewer's yeast and the same amount of lecithin, along with the 1 tablespoon of safflower oil, all in one glass of apple juice. As this detoxifies your system and rids you of acne, it should give you added energy and shiny hair. It is advisable to do this only with medical supervision, and if you can stay near a bathroom.

‡ BROWN SPOTS (LIVER SPOTS, AGE SPOTS)
The following remedies may not produce instant results. These brown spots, thought to be caused by a nutrition deficiency, took years to form. Give the remedy you use a few months to work. Then, if there's no change, change remedies.

Grate an onion and squeeze it through cheesecloth so that you have 1 teaspoon of onion juice. Mix it with 2 teaspoons of vinegar and massage the brown spots with this liquid. Do it daily—twice a day if possible—until you no longer see spots in front of your eyes.

This Israeli remedy calls for chickpeas. You may know them as garbanzo beans, ceci, or arbus. If you don't want to prepare them from scratch, buy canned chickpeas. Mash about ⅓ cupful and add a little water. Smear the paste on the brown spots and leave it there till it dries and starts crumbling off. Then wash it off completely. Do this every evening.

Once a day, take one vitamin E capsule (400 I.U.) orally. In addition, at bedtime, puncture an E capsule, squish out the oil and rub it on the brown spots, leaving it on overnight. Wear white cotton gloves to avoid messing up your linens.

A variation of this remedy is to rub on castor oil and still take the vitamin E orally.

‡ BOILS

NOTE: If pain gets progressively worse, or if you see a red streak, get professional medical attention. Don't wait! If you find the doctor's treatment is not effective, seek other medical care.

Mix 1 tablespoon of honey with 1 tablespoon of cod liver oil (Norwegian emulsified cod liver oil is nonsmelly) and glob it on the boil. Bind it with a sterile bandage. Change the dressing every 8 hours.

To draw out the waste material painlessly and quickly, add a little water to about 1 teaspoon of fenugreek powder, making it the consistency of paste. Put it on the boil and cover it with a sterile bandage. Change the dressing twice a day.

This Irish remedy requires 4 slices of bread and a cup of milk. Boil the bread and milk together until it's one big, gloppy mush. As soon as the mush is cool enough to handle, slop a glop on the boil and cover with a sterile bandage. When the glop gets cold, replace it with another warm glop. Keep redressing the boil until you've used up all 4 slices of bread. By then, the boil should have opened.

‡ WHEN THE BOIL BREAKS

The boil is at the brink of breaking when it turns red and the pain increases. When it finally does break, pus will be expelled, leaving a temporary opening in the skin. Almost magically, the pain will disappear. Boil 1 cup of water and add 2 tablespoons of lemon juice. Let it cool. Clean and disinfect the area thoroughly with the lemon water. Cover with a sterile bandage. For the next few days, two or three times a day, remove the bandage and apply a warm, wet compress, leaving it on for fifteen minutes. Redress the area with a fresh, sterile bandage.

‡ BRUISES

Grate a piece of turnip or a piece of daikon (Japanese radish). Apply the grated root to the bruise and leave it there for fifteen to thirty minutes. These two roots have been known to help clean up the internal bleeding of the bruise, preventing it from turning black and blue.

Spread a thin layer of blackstrap molasses on a piece of brown (grocery bag) paper and apply the molasses side to the bruise. Bind it in place and leave it there for hours.

Peel a banana and apply the inside of the peel to the bruise. It will lessen the pain, reduce the discoloration, and speed the healing. Bind the peel in place with a bandage.

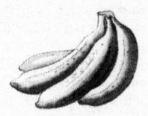

Mix 2 tablespoons of cornstarch with 1 tablespoon of castor oil. Dampen a clean white cloth and make a cornstarch/castor-oil-paste poultice. (See "Preparation Guide.") Apply the poultice to the bruise and leave it on until the damp cloth gets dry.

‡ ECZEMA
Morning and night, mix a few tablespoons of brewer's yeast with water, enough to form a paste that will cover the affected area. Gently apply it and leave it on until it dries out and crumbles off.

‡ HIVES
Hives usually disappear almost as fast and as mysteriously as they appear. If yours are hanging on, rub them with buckwheat flour. That ought to teach 'em to hang around!

Combine 3 tablespoons of cornstarch and 1 tablespoon of vinegar. Mix well and apply the paste to the hives.

‡ ITCHING (PRURITUS)

Rub the itchy area with a slice of raw potato, or grate the raw potato and use it as a poultice. (See "Preparation Guide.") It has the power to pull out the itchiness.

To stop an itch, wash the itchy part with strong rum. This remedy is from—where else?—Jamaica.

Do you have a drawstring bag made of cotton? You can sew one easily, using a white handkerchief. Fill the bag with 1 pound of uncooked oatmeal and close it tightly. Throw it in your tub as you run the warm bathwater. Then take a bath and, with the oatmeal-filled bag, gently massage the dry, itchy skin. Enjoy staying in the bath for at least 15 minutes.

‡ RECTAL ITCHING

NOTE: Rectal and genital itching may be due to an allergy, yeast overgrowth, poor hygiene, or parasites. Find the cause, and you can eliminate the problem.

For years, pumpkin seeds have been used as a folk treatment to control and prevent intestinal parasites. Buy the shelled and unsalted seeds, and eat a handful daily.

‡ GENITAL ITCHING

The Note under "Rectal Itching" also applies here.

Sprinkle cornstarch all over the area to stop the itching.

Buttermilk is known to stop the itching and help heal the area. Dip a cotton pad in some buttermilk and apply it to the problem spot.

‡ POISON IVY TEST

The white paper test will tell you if that patch of plants you just brushed up against is poison ivy. Take hold of the plant in question with a piece of white paper. Schmush the leaves, causing liquid from the plant to wet the paper. If it's poison ivy, the juice on the paper will turn black within five minutes.

‡ POISON IVY PREVENTION

The best way to avoid getting poison ivy is to know what the plant looks like and to avoid touching it. It also helps to be able to recognize jewelweed, the natural antidote. Chances are, if you know what jewelweed looks like, you'll also know what poison ivy looks like, therefore you'll have no need for jewelweed. If you do have occasion to use jewelweed, crush the leaves and stems to get the flower's juice. Apply the juice on the rash every hour throughout the day.

If possible, as soon as you think that you may have poison ivy, let cold, running water wash the plant's urushiol oil off the affected body parts. You have a very short window of opportunity to do this—about three minutes—so just hope the poison ivy patch you stepped in is near a waterfall, or a garden hose.

‡ POISON IVY RASH RELIEF

Try hard *not* to scratch the rash. (That's easy for us to say.) To help stop the itching, place ice-cold, whole-milk compresses on the affected areas. Once the rash calms down, wash the milk off with cool water. If you don't have whole milk, put ice cubes on your skin.

*　　　*　　　*

Take an oatmeal bath to ease the itching and help dry out the eruptions.

Put mashed pieces of tofu (the white, puffy, little soybean-processed pillows sold at health food stores and greengrocers) directly on the itchy areas, and bind them in place. They should help stop the itching and cool off the poison ivy flare-up.

Don't be a crab, just get one. Boil the whole crab in water, let it cool, and then use the water to wash the poison ivy area. Or, look inside the crab shell for the green stuff. Apply that green guck directly on the rash.

‡ DOING AWAY WITH THE POISON IVY PLANT

Never burn poison ivy. The plant's oil gets in the air and can be inhaled. That can be very harmful to lungs. Instead, while wearing gloves, uproot the plants and leave them on the ground to dry out in the sun. Or kill them with a solution of 3 pounds of salt in a gallon of soapy water. Spray, spray, spray the plants, and then spray them some more. Wash your garden tools thoroughly with the same solution.

Once you've gotten rid of the poison ivy and cleaned your tools, carefully take off your gloves, turn them inside out, and dispose of them. You may want to dispose of your clothes, too. Poison ivy oil may not wash out completely and can stay active for years.

‡ SHAVING RASH

Men, ever get a shaving rash, particularly on your neck? Women, all we need to say are two words: bikini area.

Puncture a vitamin E capsule, squish out the contents, and mix them with a little petroleum jelly. Then gently spread the mixture on the irritated skin.

Cornstarch makes a soothing powder for underarms and other rash-ridden areas.

‡ HEAT RASH (PRICKLY HEAT)

Make a soothing powder by browning ½ cup of regular flour in the oven.

Rub the prickly-heated area with the inside of watermelon rind.

Take a vitamin C supplement. It helps.

‡ PSORIASIS

Some people respond very well to this remedy. It's certainly worth a try. Add 1 teaspoon of sarsaparilla root (available at health food stores) to 1 cup of just-boiled water and let it steep for fifteen minutes. If it's cool enough by then, strain and saturate a white washcloth in the liquid and apply it to the trouble spot. You may need more than one washcloth, depending on the extent of the condition. If it seems to agree with you, do it morning and night for a week and watch for an improvement.

‡ SHINGLES

Did you have the chicken pox when you were a kid? Herpes zoster virus is the chicken pox virus, which is also the shingles virus, revisited. The chicken pox virus stays dormant until your immune system falls down on the job; the resulting painful, blistery flare-up is shingles.

St. John's wort is an antiviral, anti-inflammatory herb that can also strengthen the nervous system. Drink St.-John's-wort tea to help you de-stress, and gently massage the tincture directly on the affected area. Both tea and tincture are available at health food stores.

CAUTION: Be sure to check with your health professional before taking St. John's wort.

Aloe vera gel is a soothing, cooling antiseptic. You can buy a bottle of it at a health food store, or you can buy an aloe vera plant. They're inexpensive, easy to grow, and they look a lot prettier than a refrigerated bottle. Look for the aloes with the little spikes on the edge of the leaves. When using the plant, cut off the lowest leaf, then cut that leaf into 2-inch pieces. Slice one of the pieces in half and apply the gel directly on the affected area. Individually wrap the remaining pieces of the leaf in plastic wrap and keep them in the freezer. Every few hours, take a piece of leaf from the freezer and apply the gel.

Lysine may help stop the spread of the herpes zoster virus. Take lysine pills, available at health food stores (follow recommended dosage on label), or eat flounder. See the "Herpes" chapter for one man's success story. You may want to follow his lead.

CAUTION: Shingles that affect the face or forehead—anywhere near the eyes—can lead to cornea damage and/or temporary facial paralysis. Be sure to see your health professional immediately.

Make a paste of baking soda and water, and apply to the affected area for some relief.

‡ HARD-TO-HEAL SORES AND LESIONS

Some nonmalignant sores need help healing. Put pure, undiluted Concord grape juice on a sterilized cotton puff or gauze pad and apply it to the sore, binding it in place with a bandage. Do not wash the sore. Just keep the grape juice on it, changing the dressing at least once in the morning and once at night. Be patient. It may take two to three weeks for the sore to heal.

‡ SPLINTERS

Make a poultice from the grated heart of a cabbage. Apply it to the splinter and in an hour or two, it should draw the sliver out.

For real tough splinters, sprinkle salt on the splintered area, then put half a cherry tomato on it. Bind the tomato on the salted skin with a bandage and a plastic covering to keep from messing up the bed linen. Oh, we forgot to mention, you're supposed to sleep with the tomato overnight. (Now, now, fellas!) The next morning, the splinter should come right out.

‡ WARTS

Every day, apply a poultice of blackstrap molasses (see "Preparation Guide") and keep it on the wart as long as possible. You should also eat a tablespoon of molasses daily. In about two weeks, the wart should drop off without leaving a trace.

We heard about a young woman who used an old remedy. She applied regular white chalk to the wart every night.

On the sixth night, the wart fell off. She was able to chalk it up to experience.

In the morning and in the evening, rub the wart with one of the following:

a radish
juice of marigold flowers
bacon rind
oil of cinnamon
wheat germ oil
a thick paste of buttermilk and baking soda

‡ WARTS ON HAND

Boil eggs and save the water. As soon as it's cool, soak your warted hand(s) for ten minutes. Do it daily until the wart(s) disappear.

‡ PLANTAR WARTS

Plantar warts are the kind you find on the soles of the feet, usually in clusters. The wart starts as a little black dot. Don't pick it; you'll only make it spread. Instead, rub castor oil on it every night until it's history.

‡ FACIAL CARE

The first thing to ask yourself is: "What kind of skin do I have—dry, oily, combination, or normal?" If you're not sure, Heloise, the helpful hints lady, has a test you can take.

"Wash your face with shaving cream. Rinse. Wait about three hours so that your skin can revert to its regular self. Then take cigarette papers or any other thin tissue paper and press pieces of it on your face."

If it sticks, leaving an oily spot that's visible when you

hold it up to the light, you've got oily skin. If it doesn't stick, your skin is dry. If it sticks, but doesn't leave oily spots, you've got normal skin. If the papers stick on some areas, leaving oily spots, and don't stick on other areas, you have combination skin.

Now that you know what kind of skin you have, here's how to take care of it.

Always use an upward and outward motion when doing anything to one's face—whether you're washing it, doing a facial, applying makeup, or removing makeup.

When you wash your face, use tepid water. Hot or cold water may break the small capillaries—those little red squiggly veins—in your face.

It's important to wash your face two times a day or more. Washing removes dead cells, and keeps pores clean and skin texture good. The morning wash-up is necessary because of metabolic activity during the night. The night wash-up is necessary because of all the dirt that piles up during the day. Wash with a mild soap and a washcloth or cosmetic sponge, upward and outward. Now, onward . . .

NOTE: Interspersed on the following pages are recipes for masks for oily, dry, normal, and combination skin. The best time to apply a mask is at night, when you don't have to put on makeup for at least six to eight hours afterward.

It is best to apply a mask after you've taken a bath or shower, or after you've gently steamed your face, so that the pores are open.

‡ Makeup Remover for Oily Skin

Cleansers seem to be a problem for oily skin because of the high alcohol content of most makeup-removing astringents. They're usually too harsh for one's skin on a regular basis. Instead, use 1 teaspoon of powdered milk with enough warm water to give it a milky consistency. With cotton puffs, apply the liquid to your face and neck, gently rubbing it on. Once you've covered your entire face and neck, remove makeup and dirt with a tissue, again, gently. Pat dry.

‡ *Care of Oily Skin*
Many folk healers suggest drinking a strong cup of yarrow tea, which is an astringent, to cut down on skin oiliness. Use 2 teaspoons of dried yarrow (available at health food stores) in a cup of just-boiled water. Let it steep for ten minutes. Strain and drink daily.

In a blender, blend ¼ of a small eggplant (skin and all) with 1 cup of plain yogurt. Smear the mush on your face and neck (but *not* on the delicate skin around your eyes), and stay that way for twenty minutes. Rinse with tepid water. Finish this treatment with a toner—a nonalcoholic astringent like the yarrow tea in the remedy above. Fill a plastic plant mister with a cup of the tea (chamomile is also an astringent and can be used), and spray your face with it. Keep the mister in the refrigerator so you can use it to set your makeup or to freshen up.

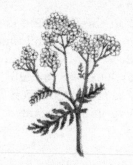

‡ *Makeup Remover for Dry Skin*
Instead of using soap and water, clean your face with whole milk. Warm 2 to 3 tablespoons of milk, add ½ tea-

spoon of castor oil, and shake well. Dunk a cotton puff (not a tissue) into the mixture and start cleaning, using upward and outward strokes. This combination of milk and oil is said to take off more makeup and city dirt than the most expensive professional cleansing products ever could. And it does it naturally, not chemically. Complete the treatment by sealing in moisture with a thin layer of castor oil.

‡ Care of Dry Skin

A leading cause of dry skin is towels. (Just checking to see if you're paying attention.)

Avocado is highly recommended for dry skin. You can use the inside of the avocado skin and massage your just-washed face and neck with it. Or, you can mix equal amounts of avocado (about ¼ cup) with sour cream. Gently rub it on the face and neck (but *not* on the delicate skin around the eyes), and leave it there for at least fifteen minutes. Rinse with tepid water. When you can no longer see a trace of the mixture, with your fingertips work the invisible oil into your skin with an upward and outward sweep, again, gently.

Another wonderful mask for dry skin is the banana mask. Look for it under "Wrinkle Prevention," later in this chapter.

‡ Care of Combination Skin

Using different masks for the dry and oily parts of your face is a real nuisance. Instead, you may want to try these treatments, good for all types of skin.

This once-a-month cleansing calls for 1 cup of uncooked oatmeal, powdered in a blender. Add 3 drops of almond oil, ½ cup of skim milk, and 1 egg white. Blend it all, then spread it on your face and neck (not around your eyes), and let it stay there for half an hour. Rinse it off with tepid water.

This papaya facial helps remove dead skin cells and allows the new skin to breathe freely. Papaya accomplishes naturally what most commercial products do chemically.

In a blender, purée a ripe, peeled papaya. Spread the fruit on your face and neck and keep it there for twenty minutes. Rinse off with tepid water. It would be good to have this facial once or twice a month, but since it's not always possible to get papaya in most areas of the country, do it whenever you can.

This mask is for everyone, all year round. It's a honey of a honey mask. Folk practitioners claim that it: helps rid the face of blemishes and blackheads; leaves you feeling refreshed and invigorated; restores weather-beaten skin; prevents skin from aging by helping it maintain the normal proportion of water in the skin. The longer we go on, the more the skin is aging. Here's how to apply the mask: Start with a clean face and neck and with your hair out of the way. Dip your fingertips in raw, unheated honey and gently spread it on your face and neck in an upward and outward motion. Leave it on for twenty minutes, then rinse it off with tepid water. It's sweet and simple . . . and sticky.

Wet your clean face and rub on a glob of petroleum jelly. Keep adding water as you thin out the layer of jelly all over your face and neck until it's no longer greasy. This inexpensive treatment is used at expensive spas because it's an effective moisturizer.

‡ SKIN AWAKENER FORMULA

One source described this apple cider vinegar treatment as "the cleansing acid that cuts through residue film and clears the way for healthful complexion breathing." Another source said, "This treatment will restore the acid covering your skin needs for protection." And still another said, "This formula is, by far, the simplest natural healer for tired skin. It gives you the glow of fresh-faced youth."

Mix 1 tablespoon of apple cider vinegar with 1 tablespoon of just-boiled water. As soon as the liquid is cool enough, apply it to the face with cotton puffs. Lydia tried it. It made her skin feel smooth and tight. Her eyes were a little teary from the strong fumes of the diluted vinegar and, for about ten minutes, she smelled like coleslaw.

Use this treatment often, at least every other day, or whenever you have a craving for coleslaw.

Some people keep a plastic plant mister filled with equal amounts of apple cider vinegar and water to spray their bodies after a shower or bath. It not only restores the acid mantle (pH balance) in the skin, it removes soap residue and hard water deposits, too.

‡ EXCELLENT EXFOLIATING FORMULA

Create a paste by mixing together ¼ cup of freshly squeezed lemon with ¼ cup extra-virgin olive oil and ½ cup of kosher (coarse) salt. Massage the paste onto the parts of your body that need exfoliating. NOT your face. It's too strong and coarse for your face. Then rinse off the mixture and feel how smooth it leaves your skin.

‡ SCARS

According to herbalist Angela Harris, you can fade away scars by applying a light film of extra-virgin, cold-pressed olive oil every day. Be consistent and be patient. It won't happen overnight.

‡ SUN-ABUSED SKIN

Soften that leathery look with this centuries-old beauty mask formula. Mix 2 tablespoons of raw honey with

2 tablespoons of flour. Add enough milk (2 to 3 tablespoons) to make it the consistency of toothpaste.

Be sure your face and neck are clean and your hair is out of the way. Smooth the paste on the face and neck. Stay clear of the delicate skin around the eyes. Leave the paste on for half an hour, rinse it off with tepid water, and pat dry.

Now you need a toner. May we make a suggestion? In a juice extractor, juice 2 cucumbers, heat to the boiling point, skim the froth off (if any), bottle the juice, and refrigerate it. Twice daily, use 1 teaspoon of juice to 2 teaspoons of water. Gently dab it on your face and neck and let it dry.

Now you need a moisturizer. Consider using a light film of extra-virgin, cold-pressed olive oil or castor oil.

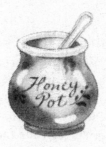

‡ FRECKLES

An old antifreckle folk remedy is to wash your face with warm beer. So, if you really want to get rid of those little brown speckles, get the warm beer and hop to it. Repeated washings several days in a row may be necessary. Also, right after the treatment, apply a light film of castor oil on your skin to prevent irritation of sensitive facial tissues.

If you're determined to do away with your freckles, bottle your own freckle remover. Get 4 medium-size dandelion leaves (either pick them yourself, or buy them at the green-grocer), rinse them thoroughly, and tear them into small pieces. Combine the leaves with 5 tablespoons of castor oil in an enamel or glass pan. Over low heat, let the mixture simmer for ten minutes. Turn off the heat, cover the pan, and let it steep for three hours. Strain the mixture into a bottle. (Don't forget to label the bottle.) Massage several drops of the oil on the befreckled area and leave it on overnight. In the morning, wash your face with tepid water. Do this daily for at least a week and watch the spots disappear.

If you're desperate to get rid of those freckles of yours, and other remedies have not worked, you may want to try this one: Take a glass of your morning urine and mix it with a tablespoon of apple cider vinegar. Add a pinch of salt and let it stand for twenty-four hours. Next, put it on the freckles for a half hour, then rinse with cool water and follow it with a thin film of castor oil. To get results, you will most likely have to do this several times. (Are you sure you really don't *want* freckles?)

Incidentally, urine has been used as an effective folk medicine for centuries. In our first folk remedy book, we wrote about a miracle acne cure using urine after everything else failed.

‡ ENLARGED PORES

So you have some enlarged pores. Think of it this way: in our 17 square feet of skin, we have about one billion pores. Percentagewise, look how few are enlarged.

To help refine those pores, put ⅓ cup of almonds into a blender and pulverize them into a powder. Add enough water to the powder to give it the consistency of paste. Rub the mixture gently across the enlarged pores from your nose outward and upward. Leave it on your face for half an hour, then rinse it off with tepid water. As a final rinse, mix ¼ cup of cool water with ¼ cup of apple cider vinegar and splash it on to tighten the pores.

You will have to treat your skin to this almond rub on a regular basis to get results.

‡ WRINKLES

We know a man who has so many wrinkles in his forehead, he has to screw his hat on. That's a lot of wrinkles. He can start to smooth them out by relaxing more, by not smoking (fact: smokers have far more wrinkles than nonsmokers), and by trying one or more of the following remedies:

Before bedtime, take extra-virgin, cold-pressed olive oil and massage the lined areas of your neck and face. Start in the center of your neck and, using an upward and outward motion, get the oil into those dry areas. Work your way up to and include your forehead. Let the oil stay on overnight. In the morning, wash with tepid, then cool, water. You may want to add a few drops of your favorite herbal essence to the olive oil, then pretend it costs $60 a bottle.

It took years to get the folds in your face, it will take time and persistence to unfold.

This is an internal approach to wrinkles. No, it doesn't mean you'll have unlined insides, it means that the nutritional value of brewer's yeast may make a difference in overcoming the external signs of time.

Start with 1 tablespoon a day of brewer's yeast in a pure fruit juice, and gradually work your way up to 2 tablespoons—a teaspoon at a time.

Some people get a gassy feeling from brewer's yeast. We were told that that means the body really needs it, and the feeling will eventually go away when the body requirements for the nutrients are met. Huh? We're not sure what it all means, but we do know that brewer's yeast contains lots of health-giving properties and it may help dewrinkle the face. Seems to us it's worth trying.

The most popular wrinkle eraser folk remedy we found requires 1 teaspoon of honey and 2 tablespoons of heavy whipping cream. Mix them together vigorously. Dip your fingertips in the mixture and, with a gentle massaging action, apply it to the wrinkles, folds, lines, creases, crinkles, whatever. Leave it on for at least half an hour, the longer the better. You'll feel it tighten on your face as it becomes a mask. When you're ready, splash it off with tepid water. By making this a daily ritual, you may become wrinkle-free.

‡ WRINKLES AROUND THE EYES
Mix the white of an egg with enough sweet cream to make it glide on your eye area. Let it stay on for at least half an hour—an hour would be twice as good. Wash it off with tepid water. The vitamins, proteins, enzymes, unsaturated fatty acids—all that great stuff—should nourish the skin cells enough to smooth out the little crinkles around the eyes. Repeat the procedure often—at least four times a week.

For those of you who haven't had eye tucks, the nightly application of castor oil on the delicate area around the eyes may prevent the need for cosmetic surgery.

‡ WRINKLE PREVENTION
To reduce the tendency to wrinkle, mash a ripe banana and add a few drops of peanut oil. Apply it to your face and neck (remember, upward and outward), and leave it on

for at least a half hour. Wash it off with tepid water. If you do this daily, or even every other day, it should make your skin softer and less likely to get lined.

If you eat oatmeal for breakfast, have we got a remedy for you. Leave some of the cooked oatmeal over. Add some vegetable oil—enough to make it spreadable—and massage it into your face and neck. Leave it on for half an hour, then wash it off with tepid water. If you want to be wrinkle-proof, you must repeat the procedure on a regular, daily basis.

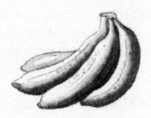

‡ LIP LINES PREVENTION
The way you may prevent those little crinkly lines around the mouth is by exercising the jaw muscle. Luckily, the jaw muscle can work the longest of all the body's muscles without getting tired. So, whistle, sing, and talk. Tongue twisters are like the aerobics of the mouth, especially ones with the "m," "b," and "p" sounds. Here are a couple to start with:

Pitter-patter, pitter-patter, rather than patter-pitter, patter-pitter.

Mother made neither brother mutter to father.

‡ DARK CIRCLES UNDER THE EYES
If you have access to fresh figs, try cutting one in half and placing the halves under your eyes. You should, of

course, lie down and relax for fifteen to thirty minutes. Okay, fig face, time to get up and gently rinse the sticky stuff off with tepid water. Dab on some peanut oil.

When figs are not in season, grate an unwaxed cucumber or a small scrubbed (preferably red) potato. Put the gratings on two gauze pads, lie down, and put them under your eyes. The rest is the same as above: rinse and dab.

‡ PUFFINESS UNDER THE EYES

We know a man who has so much puffiness under his eyes, it looks like his nose is wearing a saddle.

One of the reasons for puffiness may be an excessive amount of salt in one's diet. Salt causes water retention and water retention causes puffiness. What can be done about it? Stay away from salt. Here are some more suggestions:

When you want to look your best, set your clock an hour earlier than usual. Give yourself that extra time to depuff. Either that, or sleep sitting up so the puffs don't get a chance to form under your eyes.

Okay, you already have puffs. Wet a couple of chamomile tea bags with tepid water and put them on your problem areas. *Sit* that way for fifteen minutes.

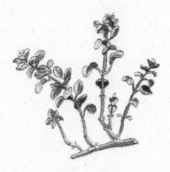

‡ ROUGH, CHAPPED, AND/OR DIRTY HANDS

For those chapped hands, try some honey. Wet your hands and shake off the water without actually drying them. Then rub some honey all over your hands. When they're completely honey-coated, let them stay that way for five minutes. (We would recommend you read the paper to pass the time, but turning the pages would definitely present problems.) Next, rub your hands as you rinse them under tepid water. Then pat your hands dry. Do this daily until you want to clap hands for your unchapped hands.

Tired of being called "lobster claw"? Take 1 teaspoon of granulated sugar in the palm of your hand and add a few drops of castor oil and enough fresh lemon juice to totally moisten the sugar. Vigorously massage your hands together for a few minutes. Rinse in tepid water and pat dry. This hand scrub should leave hands smooth and, in the process, remove stains.

One simple cleanser consists of scrubbing your hands with a palmful of dry baking soda, then rinsing with tepid water. For another, take a palmful of oatmeal, moistened with milk. Rub and rinse.

This folk remedy for rough, chapped, and soiled hands is a favorite among farmers. In a bowl combine about ¼ cup of cornmeal, 1 tablespoon of water, and enough apple cider vinegar to make the mixture the consistency of a loose paste. Rub this mildly abrasive mixture all over your hands for ten minutes. Rinse with tepid water and pat dry. This treatment not only can remove dirt, it can also soften, soothe, and heal the hands.

‡ CLAMMY HANDS

In a basin, combine ½ gallon of water with ½ cup of alcohol and bathe your hands in the mixture. After a few minutes, rinse your hands with cool water and pat dry. This is especially useful for clammy-palmed politicians on the campaign trail.

‡ FINGERNAILS

If you're having problems with breaking, splitting, and thin nails, you may need to supplement your diet with a vitamin B complex and zinc sulfate (follow the directions on the bottle for the dosage), along with garlic—raw and/or supplements.

The following folk remedies for strengthening fingernails can help if they're in addition to a well-balanced diet.

Daily, soak your fingers for ten minutes in any one of the oils listed:

- warm olive oil
- warm sesame-seed oil
- warm wheat germ oil

As you wipe off the oil, give your nails a mini-massage from top to bottom.

If your nails are very brittle, use a juice extractor to juice parsnip—enough for ½ cup at a time. Drink parsnip juice at least once a day. Be patient for results. Give it a couple of weeks or more.

While tapping your nails on a table can be very annoying to people around you, it is very good for your nails. The more you tap, the faster they will grow. You may need long nails to defend yourself from those annoyed people around you.

‡ NICOTINE NAILS

If your nails are cigarette stained, we'll tell you how to bleach them back to normal if you promise to stop smoking, okay? Now then, rub half a lemon over your nails. Then remove the lemon's pulp and, with the remaining rind, concentrate on one nail at a time, rubbing each one until it looks nice and pink.

NOTE: If you have citrus juice on your skin and you go in the sun, your skin may become permanently mottled. Be sure to wash the lemon juice off before you go outdoors.

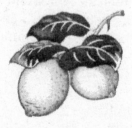

‡ STAINED NAILS

Want natural, healthy-looking, pinkish nails? Gaby Nigai, co-owner of Ellegee Nail Salon in New York City, offers this good advice: Stop staining them with colored nail polish. From now on, first wear a protein-based coat under nail polish to protect your nails from the polish's color pigments, which cause the staining and oxidation.

To get rid of the stains, toss 2 denture-cleansing tablets into ¼ cup of water. Soak your fingertips in the solution for about fifteen minutes. If your nails are not as stain-free as you had hoped, gently brush them with a nailbrush. Rinse and dry.

*   *   *

Put tooth-whitening paste on a toothbrush and gently distribute the paste on your nails. Leave it on for about fifteen minutes; brush as you rinse off the paste. Then dry.

NOTE: It may take several tries, day after day, before the stains are completely gone. Work at it; your appearance is worth it!

‡ ELBOWS AND KNEES

Take the skin from half an avocado and rub the inside of it against the rough areas of your elbows and/or knees. Keep rubbing. Don't wash off the area until bedtime.

Rest your elbows in grapefruit halves to get rid of alligator skin. Make yourself as comfortable as possible and keep your elbows in the citrus fruit for at least a half hour.

‡ HELPFUL GROOMING HINTS

‡ Instant, Temporary Eye Tuck

You can smooth out the lined area under your eyes. This show biz trick is fine for a photo session but not for anything that lasts longer than three hours.

Take an egg white and beat it frothy. Then, with a fine brush—an eyeliner brush, for example—paint the under-the-eye area. The secret of success here is to paint as thin and as even an egg white layer as possible. As you allow it to dry, you'll notice how the area tightens. Use liquid makeup on top and instead of rubbing it on, gently pat on the makeup.

As soon as you wash off the egg white, lubricate the area with castor oil to help undo the drying effects of the egg.

‡ Face Relaxer

Before applying your evening makeup, take time to get the day's tension out of your face. Here's how: Lie down with your feet up. Take a wine bottle cork and put it between your teeth. Don't bite down on it; encircle it with your lips. Stay that way for ten minutes of easy breathing and lovely thoughts.

After the ten minutes have flown by, your *face* should be smoother and more receptive to makeup. And *you* should be refreshed and more receptive to having a fun evening.

‡ Makeup Remover

No makeup remover? Use whipped sweet butter or a vegetable shortening like Crisco, instead. (Doesn't this sound like it's right out of a *Cosmopolitan* magazine list of "sleep over" suggestions?)

Whatever makeup remover you use, keep it on your eyes and face for at least thirty seconds so that it has a chance to sink in and make it easier to gently rub off the makeup.

‡ Paint Remover for Skin

A little vegetable oil should clean off your paint-bespeckled face and arms without torturing your skin.

‡ Bandage Remover

When you're wearing a bandage that's not "ouchless," saturate it with vegetable oil so that you can remove it painlessly.

‡ Enrich Your Night Cream

According to cosmetics expert Adrien Arpel, "To transform a skimpy night cream into an enriched vitamin skin treat, add ⅛ teaspoon of liquid vitamin C and the contents of a 100 I.U. vitamin E capsule to 4 ounces of ordinary night cream."

‡ Double-Chin Prevention

Do a simple yoga exercise called "the lion." Start firming up the throat muscles under the chin. The entire exercise consists of sticking your tongue out and down as far as it will go. Do it dozens of times throughout the day, in your car, watching TV, while doing the dishes, or waiting for your computer to boot up.

It's possible you'll see an improvement in your chin line within a few days.

‡ Nail File Substitute

When you need an emery board and nobody has one, chances are somebody will have a matchbook. File down a jagged-edged fingernail with the rough, striking part of the matchbook.

‡ Polish Primer

Wipe your unpolished fingernails with vinegar to clean and prime the surfaces for nail polish. This treatment will help the polish stay on longer.

‡ Manicure Protection

Use a toothbrush and toothpaste to clean office-type stains (carbon, ink, etc.) off your fingertips without damaging your manicure.

‡ Toweling Off

Towels made of 100 percent cotton will dry you faster and more thoroughly than towels made of blended fibers.

‡ Mirror, Mirror, in the Bathroom

Clean the mirror with shaving cream, and it will prevent it from fogging up for several weeks. If you didn't do the shaving cream bit, after a shower or bath use a hair dryer to unfog the steamed-up mirror.

‡ *Pleasing Tweezing*

If you can't stand the pain of tweezing your eyebrows, numb the area first by putting an ice cube on for a few seconds.

If you don't need to go so far as to numb the area, but just want to have an easy time of it, tweeze right after a warm shower. The hairs come out more willingly then.

‡ *Perfume Pick-Me-Up*

Dowse a small natural sponge with your favorite perfume and put it in a plastic sandwich bag in your pocketbook. During or after a hard day at the office, moisten the sponge with some cold water and dab it behind your ears and knees, in your elbows, and on your wrists to give you a refreshed feeling.

‡ Sleep

‡ INSOMNIA

You know you have insomnia if you can't sleep even when it's time to get up.

A popular folk remedy for insomnia is counting sheep. We heard about a garment manufacturer who had trouble sleeping. Not only did he count sheep, he sheared them, combed the wool, had it spun into yarn, woven into cloth, made into suits, distributed them in town, watched as they didn't sell, had them returned, and lost thousands on the deal. That's why he had trouble sleeping in the first place. We have some other folk remedies to help him and you get a good night's sleep.

In England, it is believed that a good night's sleep will be ensured if you lie in bed with your head to the north and your feet to the south.

Nutmeg can act as a sedative. Steep ½ of a crushed nutmeg (not more than that) in hot water for ten minutes and drink it a half hour before bedtime. If you don't like the taste of it, you can use nutmeg oil externally. Rub it on your forehead.

Try drinking a glass of pure, warmed grapefruit juice. If you need it sweetened, use raw honey.

This Silva Mind Control process seems to zzzzzzz. Where was I? Oh yes, once you're in bed, completely relax. Lightly close your eyes. Now picture a blackboard. Take a piece of imaginary chalk and draw a circle. Within the circle, draw a square and put the number 99 in the square. Erase the number 99. Be careful you don't erase the sides of the square. Replace 99 with 98. Then erase 98 and replace it with 97, then 96, 95, 94, etc. You should fall asleep long before you get Bingo!

Macrobiotic leader Michio Kushi says that when you can't sleep, put a cut, raw onion under your pillow. No, you don't cry yourself to sleep. There's something in the onion that scurries you off to dreamland.

We have another version of this remedy that's as effective, and won't mess up your pillow or linens. Cut a yellow onion in chunks and place it in a glass jar. Put the cover on the jar, and keep it on your night table. When you can't fall asleep, or when you wake up and can't fall back asleep, open the jar and take a deep whiff or two of the onion. Close the jar, lie back, think lovely thoughts, and within fifteen minutes, zzzzzzz.

A relaxing bath may help you fall asleep. Before you take your bath, prepare a cup of sleep-inducing herb tea to drink as soon as you get out of the tub. Use chamomile, sage, or fresh ginger tea. Then take a bath using any one or a combination of the following herbs: lavender, marigold, passionflower, and/or rosemary. (See "Preparation Guide.") All the herbs should be available at health food stores.

By the time you finish your bath and the tea, you should be wound down and ready to doze off.

A gem therapist told us about the power of a diamond. Set in a silver ring, it supposedly prevents insomnia. The therapist also said that wearing a diamond, in any setting, protects the wearer from nightmares. Well, there you have one of the best arguments for getting engaged.

* * *

A glass of elderberry juice, at room temperature, is thought of as a sleep inducer. You can get pure elderberry concentrate at health food stores. Just dilute it, drink it, and hit the hay.

According to the record (please don't ask us which one), King George III was plagued with insomnia until a physician prescribed a hop pillow. Hops have been known to have a tranquilizing effect on people. Lupulin, an active ingredient in hops, has been used to treat a variety of nervous disorders.

Buy or sew together a little muslin or fine white cotton bag. Fill it with hops and tack it to your pillow. Change the hops once a month.

It is believed by some that the hop pillow will be a more effective sedative if you lightly spray it with alcohol.

You may want to try placing a pillow, which is filled with flaxseeds, *on* your eyes to help you fall asleep. Many health food stores carry them, and you can find them online at health-supplies sites. The eye pillow applies just enough pressure to the eyes and orbits to help you relax.

A naturopath we met has had great success in treating severe insomniac patients with goat's milk. He recommends they drink 6 ounces before each meal and 6 ounces before bedtime. Within a week, he has seen patients go from two hours sleep a night, to sleeping eight restful hours of sleep night after night. Some supermarkets as well as health food stores sell goat's milk.

Galen, a great Greek physician, was able to cure his own insomnia by eating lots of lettuce in the evening. Lettuce has lactucarium, a calming agent. The problem with eating lots of lettuce is that it's a diuretic. So, while it may help you fall asleep, you may have to get up in the middle of the night to go to the bathroom.

Worried about not being able to fall asleep? Okay then, don't let yourself go to sleep. That's right, try to stay awake. Sleep specialists call this technique "paradoxical intent." When we were children and our father used it on us, we precociously called it "reverse psychology." So, take the worry out of trying to go to sleep, and try hard to stay awake. You'll be asleep in no time.

Keep the room temperature cool and your feet warm. Wear socks to bed, or rest your feet on a hot water bottle. According to a study done at the Chronobiology and Sleep Laboratory in Basel, Switzerland, sleepiness is caused by a drop in core body temperature. That happens as your body heat slowly dissipates through dilated blood vessels in the feet. Aside from falling asleep faster, warm feet are more comfortable for you and your bedmate.

‡ NIGHTMARE PREVENTION

Lightly sprinkle essence of anise (available at health food stores) on your pillow so that you inhale the scent as soon as you lie down. It is said to give one "happy" dreams, restful sleep, and an oil-stained pillowcase.

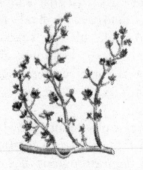

‡ SNORE STOPPER

Lightly tickle the snorer's throat and the snoring should stop. Of course the laughing may keep you up.

‡ SNORING

Actually, *snoring* is not a laughing matter. Chronic snoring, that is, snoring every night and loudly, may be the start of a serious condition known as sleep apnea. Apnea is Latin for "without breath." During the night, the windpipe keeps blocking as the throat relaxes and closes, making it difficult to breathe. After holding one's breath for an unnatural amount of time (anywhere from ten seconds to a couple of minutes), the snore comes as the person gasps for air. The person partially awakens each time it happens, and it can happen dozens and dozens of times during the night, without the person realizing it. The interrupted sleep causes that person to be tired all day. It can then be dangerous being behind the wheel of a car, operating heavy machinery, or just crossing a street. Aside from the daytime accident aspect, sleep apnea may lead to high blood pressure, heart problems, and stroke.

If you think that you may have sleep apnea, ask your doctor to recommend a sleep specialist right away. There are sleep clinics throughout the country.

Meanwhile, all snorers can minimize or completely eliminate their nighttime noise three ways:
- *If you smoke, stop!* Let your smoker's inflamed, swollen throat tissues heal.
- *If you drink, don't!* Alcoholic beverages relax the respiratory system muscles, making it harder to breathe and, in turn, promote snoring.
- *If you're overweight, trim down!* Fat deposits at the base of the tongue contribute to the blocking of an already-clogged airway. Also, wait a couple of hours

after you've eaten before going to sleep to avoid additional congestion.

You may want to try sewing a tennis ball on the back of the snorer's pajama top or nightgown. This prevents the snorer from sleeping on his or her back, which prevents snoring.

‡ SLEEPWALKING

A Russian professor who studied sleepwalkers recommended that a piece of wet carpeting be placed right by the sleepwalker's bed. In most cases, the sleepwalker awoke the second his or her feet stepped on the wet carpet.

‡ Sore Throats

Some sore throats are caused by allergies, smoking, post-nasal drip, yeast overgrowth, and varying severities of bacterial invasion into your throat tissues. You may need a health professional to help you determine the cause.

Many sore throats are caused by a mild viral infection that attacks when your resistance is low.

If you have a sore throat right now, think about your schedule. Chances are, you've been pushing yourself like crazy, running around, and keeping later hours than usual.

If you take it easy, get a lot of rest, flush your system by drinking nondairy liquids, and stay away from heavy foods, the remedies we suggest will be much more effective.

NOTE: The presence of enlarged lymph nodes below the angles of the jaw, and fever, as well as continuation of throat soreness suggest that you should seek medical attention.

‡ SORE THROATS IN GENERAL

Prepare chamomile tea. As soon as it cools enough for you to handle, soak a towel, preferably white, in the tea, wring it out, and apply it to the throat. As soon as it gets cold, reheat the tea, redip the towel, and reapply it. The chamomile will help draw out the soreness; the heat will relax some of the tension built up in that area.

According to a gem therapist, yellow amber worn around the neck will protect against sore throats. If you already have a sore throat, it is said that the electric powers of this fossilized, golden resin will help cure it.

*   *   *

In all good conscience, Joan could not talk about sore throat remedies without including her sure-cure, even though it's in our first folk remedy book.

Add 2 teaspoons of apple cider vinegar to 1 glass of luke-warm water. Gargle a mouthful and spit it out, then swallow a mouthful. Gargle a mouthful, spit it out, then swallow a mouthful. Notice a pattern forming here? Keep going that way until you finish the glass of vinegar water. Repeat the procedure every hour. Joan has never had to do it more than two or three hours in a row for the sore throat to be history.

Prepare a carrot poultice (see "Preparation Guide") with a large, grated carrot. Put the poultice around your throat. For warmth, put on top of the poultice a washcloth that has been dipped in hot water and wrung out. To keep the heat in, cover it all with a towel or wide Ace bandage. If it seems to soothe your throat, redip the washcloth in hot water as soon as it gets cold.

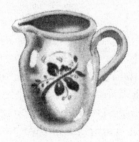

‡ STREP THROAT CAUSES

Do you have a dog or a cat? If you do and you're troubled by frequent bouts of strep throat, have a veterinarian examine the animal for streptococci. Once your pet is free of the bacteria, chances are you will be, too, after treatment by your health professional.

*　　*　　*

If you participate in oral sex, have your partner's part checked. It may help you find out why you keep getting strep throat. . . .

‡ LARYNGITIS/HOARSENESS

Rest your vocal cords as much as possible. If you have to talk, talk in a normal voice, letting the sound come from your diaphragm instead of your throat. DON'T WHISPER! Whispering tightens the muscles of your voice box, and puts more stress on your vocal cords than does talking in your normal voice.

See the apple cider vinegar remedy in "Sore Throats in General" above. After seven hours and seven doses of the vinegar and water, and a good night's sleep, there should be a major improvement.

If your cold seemed to settle in your throat in the form of hoarseness and congestion, peel and mince an entire bulb of garlic. Cover all the little pieces with raw honey and let it stand for two hours. Take a teaspoon of the honey/garlic mixture every hour. Just swallow it down without chewing the garlic. That way you won't have garlic on your breath.

Grate radishes and squeeze them through cheesecloth to get radish juice. Let a teaspoon of the juice slide down your throat every half hour.

This is a popular Russian remedy for what they call "singer's sore throat." It promises to restore the singer's voice to normal in a single day.
Take ½ cup of anise seeds and 1 cup of water and boil them slowly for fifty minutes. Strain out the seeds, then stir ¼ cup of raw honey into the anise-seed water and add 1 tablespoon of cognac.

DOSE: 1 tablespoon every half hour.

Incidentally, you don't have to be a singer to try this formula.

‡ TONSILLITIS

NOTE: If you keep getting tonsillitis, your immune system needs to be evaluated and treated. Be aware that untreated bacterial tonsillitis may have serious consequences, including rheumatic fever, scarlet fever, or even kidney disease (nephritis).

Bake a medium-size banana in its skin for thirty minutes at 350 degrees. Peel and mash the juicy banana, adding 1 tablespoon of extra-virgin, cold-pressed olive oil. Spread the mush on a clean white cloth and apply it to the neck. Leave it on for one half hour in the morning and one half hour in the evening.

Juice garlic cloves (see "Preparation Guide") so that you have 1 tablespoon of the fresh juice. Add the juice and 2 ounces of dried sage to 1 quart of water in a glass or enamel pot. Cover the pot and bring the mixture to a boil. As soon as it starts to boil, turn off the heat and let it stand until it's lukewarm. Strain the solution.

DOSE: Drink ½ cup of this sage-garlic tea every two hours. Gargle ½ cup every hour until the condition is better.

The holistic health professionals we talked to believe that tonsils should not be removed unless it's absolutely necessary. They function as armed guards, destroying harmful bacteria that enter through the mouth. Asian medicine practitioners feel that when tonsils are unable to fulfill this function, it's not that the tonsils should be taken out, it's that the body's immune system needs to be strengthened.

‡ Sprains, Strains, Pains, and Muscle Stiffness

According to Dr. Ray C. Wunderlich, Jr., of the Wunderlich Center for Nutritional Medicine in St. Petersburg, Florida, as soon as you get a sprain, take large amounts of enzymes hourly, in the form of fresh vegetable juices and/or bromelain, papaya, and pancreatic supplements (available at health food stores). The sooner you start taking enzymes, the better! Then read on to decide what to do next.

For our first folk remedy book, we questioned medical professionals about what to do for a sprain, and we reported the consensus, which we feel should be repeated here:

During the first twelve hours after the injury, starting as soon as possible, apply an ice-cold water compress to the area to reduce the swelling caused by the sprain. Leave the ice pack on for twenty minutes, then take it off for twenty minutes. Extend the twelve hours of cold compresses to twenty-four hours if it seems necessary. It would be wise to seek medical attention to make sure the sprain is nothing more than a sprain and not a fractured, chipped, or dislocated bone.

Since the publication of that book, we've heard about other remedies that have worked wonderfully well. For instance . . .

Immediately dunk the sprained area into a basin of very hot water. Keep the water hot, not scalding, just hot, by adding more hot water during this ten-minute soaking period. Then transfer the sprained area to a basin of ice-cold water and keep it there for five minutes. Next, bind the area with a wet bandage and cover the wet one with a dry bandage.

✻　　✻　　✻

Warm a cupful of apple cider vinegar, saturate a wash-cloth with it, and apply the cloth to the sprain for five minutes every hour.

Take the peel of an orange and apply it to the sprained area—the white spongy side on the skin—and bind it in place with a bandage. It should reduce the swelling of a sprain.

Add 1 tablespoon of cayenne pepper to 2 cups of apple cider vinegar and bring it to a slow boil in an enamel or glass saucepan. Bottle the liquid and use it on sprains, pains, and sore muscles.

Grate ginger and squeeze the grated ginger through cheesecloth, getting as much juice as you can. Measure the amount of ginger juice and add an equal amount of sesame oil. Mix it thoroughly and massage it on your painful parts.

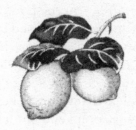

This remedy is said to be particularly effective for a charley horse (muscle stiffness). Vigorously scrub 3 small lemons, 2 small oranges, and 1 small grapefruit. (If you can get organic produce, do so.) Cut up the 6 fruits and put them into a blender—peel and all. Add 1 teaspoon of cream of tartar and blend. Store the mixture in a covered jar in the refrigerator. Take 2 tablespoons of the concoction with 2 tablespoons of water twice a day—first thing in the morning and right before bedtime.

*　　*　　*

Add 1 teaspoon of catnip to 1 cup of just-boiled water and steep for five minutes. Saturate a washcloth with the catnip tea and apply it to the sprained area to reduce swelling. When the washcloth gets to be room temperature, resaturate the cloth in the heated liquid and reapply it.

Comfrey is getting more and more popular among professional athletes and their smart coaches. This herb helps speed up the healing process and relieve the pain of pulled tendons and ligaments, strains, sprains, broken bones, and tennis elbow.

Use a comfrey poultice (see "Preparation Guide") on the sprained area, changing it every two to three hours. Also, drink 2 to 4 cups of comfrey a day. Comfrey roots and leaves and comfrey tea bags are available at health food stores.

‡ TENNIS ELBOW (SEE COMFREY REMEDY, ABOVE)

‡ RECURRENT–SPRAIN PREVENTION

This applies mostly to athletes and dancers who keep spraining the same weakened parts of their bodies. Before a warm-up session, saturate a washcloth with hot water and apply it to your vulnerable area for ten to fifteen minutes. In other words, preheat the trouble spot before you work out.

‡ Stings and Bites

In our first folk remedy book we listed the most effective pain and swelling reducers for stings and bites: raw onion or potato, wet soap, wet salt, commercial toothpaste, dampened tobacco, vitamin E, raw honey, diluted ammonia, meat tenderizer, mud, or equal parts of vinegar mixed with lemon juice.

We now add to the above list a paste made with water and baking soda. It can help draw out the heat of a sting, reduce the redness, inhibit the swelling, and take the itch out of a bite. Every half hour alternate the baking soda paste with ice on the stung or bitten area.

Wheat germ oil helps soothe a sting. Every half hour alternate the wheat germ oil with ice on the stung area.

‡ THROAT STINGS

Being stung in the throat is a revolting thought that seems impossible. It's a rare occurrence but it has and can happen, especially when eating fresh fruit. Quickly mix 2 teaspoons of salt in some water and gargle. Keep gargling. The salt water will draw out the poison and, most important, it will stop the area from swelling.

‡ TICKS

This is not a pleasant thought but a remarkable remedy. If a tick has embedded itself in your skin, take clear fingernail polish and drip two drops on the insect. It will release its grasp and back out. Just wipe it off your skin.

‡ MOSQUITO AND GNAT BITE PREVENTION

Remember how, when you were a child and got bitten up by mosquitoes, your mother would say, "That's because you're so sweet." There may be something to it. Experiments were conducted with people who completely eliminated white sugar and alcoholic beverages from their diets. They were surrounded by mosquitoes and gnats. Not only were those people *not* bitten, the insects didn't even bother to land on them. Conclusion: If you're sugar-free, it's so long mosquitoes, and gnuts to gnats!

Mosquitoes have been known to stay away from people whose systems have a high amount of vitamin B_1 (thiamine). Before you go to a mosquito-infested area, eat foods that are rich in B_1: sunflower seeds, brewer's yeast, Brazil nuts, and fish.

Keep geraniums on porches and other places you like to sit. The potted geraniums keep mosquitoes away.

If you dread mosquito bites more than you mind smelling from garlic, have we got a remedy for you. Rub garlic over all your exposed body parts before reaching a mosquito-infested area. Mosquitoes will not come near you. They hate garlic. Garlic is to mosquitoes what kryptonite is to Superman.

Biologist Eldon L. Reeves of the University of California tested garlic extract on five species of mosquitoes. The garlic got 'em. Not one mosquito survived.

‡ FOUR-LEGGED ANIMAL BITES

If you're bitten by an animal get medical attention immediately!

* * *

If you are going on safari, or will be away from professional health care for days at a time, take fresh, hot red peppers, an enamel pan, sesame oil, and clean white handkerchiefs.

After being bitten by an animal, this remedy has been known to counteract rabies. Use it *only* if professional medical help is not available.

Sauté a few pieces of a hot red pepper with some sesame oil in the pan. When the pepper is wilted, put it on a handkerchief and apply it directly to the bite. When the oily, wilted piece of pepper dries up, replace it with another piece of oily, wilted pepper. Keep repeating this procedure for three days, at which time the toxins should be out of your system.

‡ RATTLESNAKE BITE PREVENTION

When Texas panhandlers camped out under the stars, they put their lariat ropes in a circle on the ground, and put their sleeping bags in the middle of it. It seems to be a known fact in the Texas panhandle that rattlesnakes will not crawl across a rope.

My luck, a nearsighted rattler would be passing by and fall in love with the rope.

‡ Stop Smoking

Surely you know that smoking can cause, contribute to, or worsen backaches, bronchitis, cataracts, emphysema, gum problems, hangovers, infertility, osteoporosis, phlebitis, sleep disorders including sleep apnea, sore throats, tinnitus, ulcers, varicose veins, endometriosis, heartburn, diverticulosis . . . And that's just for starters. Cigarette smoking has been linked to every serious disease. We'll spare you the statistics from the American Heart Association, the American Lung Association, and the American Cancer Society on the estimated number of Americans who die before they reach retirement age because of smoking.

All the talk about sickness and premature death doesn't seem to motivate smokers—especially teenagers or young adults—to stop. Dr. James Duke has a wake-up call. He likes to remind young smokers that the habit hits men in the penis and women in the face. "Smoking damages the blood vessels that supply the penis, so men who smoke have an increased risk of impotence. Smoking also damages the capillaries in women's faces, which is why women (and men) smokers develop wrinkles years before nonsmokers."

Ready to stop smoking? Hopefully the following suggestions will help make it easier.

‡ WAYS TO HELP YOU QUIT

Make a list of all the reasons you want to quit. You may want to divide the list into "short-term reasons," like: wanting to be more kissable; and "long-term reasons," like: wanting to walk your daughter down the aisle at her wedding. Keep the list handy and refer to it each time you're about to give in and smoke.

A professor of behavioral medicine suggests that when the

craving comes over you, pick up a pen instead of a cigarette, and write a letter to loved ones, telling them why smoking is more important than they are. Tell them how you choose to die young and how you'll miss sharing in their happiness. Apologize for having to have someone take care of you when you're no longer well enough to take care of yourself. Got the picture? These, hopefully, *unfinished* letters may give you the strength to pass up a cigarette one more time, each time, until you no longer have the horrible craving to smoke.

Nobel laureate professor of chemistry Dr. Linus Pauling suggests you eat an orange whenever you have the urge to smoke. The Outspan Organization in Britain conducted experiments with smokers and oranges. The results were impressive. By the end of three weeks, the orange-eating cigarette smokers smoked 79 percent fewer cigarettes than they ordinarily would have; 20 percent kicked the habit completely. It seems that eating citrus fruit has a kick that's similar to smoking a cigarette. Incidentally, the Outspan Organization recommends that when you take a piece of orange instead of smoking a cigarette, first suck the juice out and then eat the pulp.

To many smokers, the thought of smoking a cigarette after they've had a citrus drink is unpleasant. If you feel that way, *good!* Carry a small bottle of citrus juice with you and whenever you feel like lighting up, take a swig of the juice. Since each cigarette robs your body of between 25 and 100 mg of vitamin C, the juice will help replenish it as well as keep you from smoking.

To help cleanse your system of nicotine, and to help prevent tumors from forming, take ½ teaspoon of red clover tincture (available at health food stores) three times a day. Drinking a cup of red clover tea once or twice a day may also help.

To help detoxify your liver, drink 2 cups of milk thistle seed tea before every meal. In case you're worried about gaining weight now that you're not going to be smoking, these 6 cups of tea before meals may help you cut down on the amount of food you eat.

Marjoram tea (available at health food stores) can help you be a former cigarette smoker. The tea makes your throat very dry and so smoking will not be nearly as pleasurable. Marjoram is naturally sweet; nothing needs to be added to it. Have a cup of tea when you would ordinarily have your first cigarette of the day. Try ½ cup after that whenever you have an uncontrollable urge to smoke.

According to some Chinese herbalists, magnolia-bark tea is effective in curbing the desire to light up. You might want to alternate between magnolia-bark and marjoram (above) teas.

Dr. James Duke smoked three packs of unfiltered, king-size cigarettes a day, until the day he quit—cold turkey. That was close to three decades ago. According to Dr. Duke, carrots helped him quit. He would munch on raw carrots instead of puffing on a cigarette. "If cigarettes are cancer sticks," says Dr. Duke, "carrots are anticancer sticks." He explains that carotenoids, the chemical relatives of vitamin A, help prevent cancer, especially if the carotenoids come from carrots or other whole foods rather than from capsules. Carrots also help lower cholesterol levels.

Buy a package of baby carrots and munch on them throughout the day.

Apricots are rich in beta-carotene, potassium, boron, iron, and silica. Not only do they help prevent cancer, they are also good for the heart, for promoting estrogen in postmenopausal women, for preventing fatigue and infection, and for healthy skin, hair, and nails. Apricots are especially good for helping to minimize the long-term potential harm caused by nicotine. Start eating a few dried apricots a day and continue eating them even as a nonsmoker. Buy the unsulfured dried apricots. Sulfur (sulfite) preservatives can produce allergic reactions, especially in asthmatics. Also, the long-term accumulation of sulfites can cause unhealthy conditions.

In addition to carrots and apricots (above), unsalted, raw sunflower seeds are another wonderful munchie. Tobacco releases stored sugar (glycogen) from the liver and it perks up one's brain. Sunflower seeds provide that same mental lift. Tobacco has a sedative effect that tends to calm a person down. Sunflower seeds also stabilize the nerves because they contain oils that are calming, and B-complex vitamins that help nourish the nervous system. (Maybe that's why baseball players are eating them during a game.) Tobacco increases the output of adrenal gland hormones, which reduces the allergic reaction of smokers. Sunflower seeds do the same.

Keep in mind that the seeds are fairly high in fat, so don't overdo it. Consider buying sunflower seeds with shells. The shelling process will slow down your consumption of the seeds.

‡ THE DREADED WITHDRAWAL TIME

During the worst time, the dreaded week or two of withdrawal, push yourself to exercise—walk, swim, bowl, play table tennis, clean your house, do gardening, play with a yo-yo. *Keep moving.* It will make you feel better. It will help prevent weight gain. Incidentally, gaining five to ten pounds because you stopped smoking is worth it when you consider the health risks of smoking. But if you follow these suggestions, and also start eating the foods in the "Sensational Six Superfoods" chapter, you may stop smoking and *not* gain any weight:

1. *Be kind to yourself and don't place temptation in your face.* Do not frequent bars or other places where people smoke-smoke-smoke. Hang out at places where smoking is *not* permitted: movie theaters, museums, the library, houses of worship, adult education courses at schools.

2. Figure out how much money you'll save a year by not smoking. Decide on exactly what you want to do with that money—special treat(s) for yourself—and actually put that money away in a safe each time you *don't* buy a pack of cigarettes when you ordinarily would have.

‡ ONCE YOU QUIT . . .

A nicotine-dependency researcher reported that nicotine causes smokers to process caffeine two and a half times faster than nonsmokers. So, once you quit smoking, and the nicotine is washed out of your system, you'll need only about a third as much coffee to get the same *buzz* you got from drinking coffee while still smoking. The same goes for alcoholic beverages. Take into consideration that you'll get drunk faster without nicotine in your body. Think of the additional money you'll be saving on coffee and booze.

‡ CLEARING THE AIR

If cigarette smokers are at your home or office and you don't want to ask them not to smoke, place little saucers of vinegar around the room in inconspicuous spots. The vinegar will absorb the smell of tobacco smoke.

Burning candles add atmosphere to a room and absorb cigarette smoke at the same time.

‡ Teeth, Gums, and Mouth

‡ TOOTHACHE

Toothache? Until you get to the dentist for the drilling, filling, and billing, try one or more of these remedies to ease the pain.

Prepare a cup of chamomile tea and saturate a white washcloth in it. Wring it out, then apply it to your cheek or jaw—the outside area of your toothache. As soon as the cloth gets cold, redip it and reapply it. This chamomile compress should draw out the pain before it's time to reheat the tea.

Soak your feet in hot water. Dry them thoroughly, then rub them vigorously with bran. No, this didn't get mixed into the wrong category. We were told this is a Cherokee Indian remedy for a toothache.

Whenever the subject of toothaches came up in our home, we would prompt our dad to tell the "pig fat" story. He would begin by telling us that when he was a teenager, he had dental work done and it was on a Thursday. Late that night, there was swelling and pain from the work the dentist did. In those days, dentists were not in their offices on Friday, and the thought of waiting till Monday was out of the question because the pain was so severe. Friday morning, our grandmother went to the nonkosher butcher in the neighborhood and bought a piece of pig fat. She brought it into the house (something she had *never* done before, since she kept a strictly kosher home), heated it up, and put the melted fat on a white handkerchief, which she then placed on Daddy's cheek. Within a few minutes, the swelling went down and the pain vanished. Right about now in the telling of this story, our dad would get up and demonstrate how he danced around the room, celebrating his freedom from pain.

Recently, we've come across another version of that toothache remedy (we promise, no more stories). Take a tiny slice of pig fat and place it between the gum and cheek, directly on the sore area. Keep it there for fifteen minutes, or however long it takes for the pain to subside. The dance afterward is optional.

Make a cup of stronger-than-usual sage tea. If your teeth are not sensitive to "hot," hold the hot tea in your mouth for half a minute, then swallow and take another mouthful. Keep doing this until you finish the cup of tea and, hopefully, have no more pain.

Take 50 to 100 mg of niacin to relieve the pain of a toothache. You may get the "niacin flush." Don't worry. The redness and tingling will disappear in a short while, hopefully along with the toothache.

‡ CAVITY PREVENTION

To avoid being "bored" to tears by the dentist, eat a little cube of cheddar, Monterey Jack, or Swiss cheese right after eating cavity-causing foods. It seems that cheese reduces bacterial acid production, which causes decay. Peanuts also help prevent tooth decay. They can be eaten at the end of the meal, instead of right after each cavity-causing food. We thank the National Institute of Dental Research for this information.

Tea is rich in fluoride, which resists tooth decay. Some Japanese tea drinkers believe it helps fight plaque. Take tea and see. You may want to try Kukicha tea. It's tasty, relaxing, caffeine-free, and available at health food stores or Asian markets. Incidentally, you can use the same Kukicha tea bag three or four times.

Blackstrap molasses contains an ingredient that seems to inhibit tooth decay. Sunflower seeds are also supposed to inhibit tooth decay. Have a tablespoon of molasses in water and/or a handful of shelled, raw, unsalted sunflower seeds daily. Be sure to rinse thoroughly with water after the molasses.

‡ CLEAN YOUR TOOTHBRUSH

Dissolve a tablespoon of baking soda in a glass of warm water and soak your toothbrush in it overnight. Rinse it in the morning and notice how clean it looks and feels.

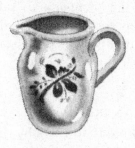

‡ THROW AWAY YOUR TOOTHBRUSH

Bacteria from your mouth nestle in the bristles of your toothbrush and can reinfect you with whatever you have—a cold sore, a cold, the flu, or a sore throat. As soon as symptoms appear, throw away your toothbrush. Use a new one for a few days, then throw that one away, and use another new one. If you want to be super-cautious, use a brand-new toothbrush as soon as you're all better.

‡ GUM PROBLEMS (PYORRHEA)

Brush your teeth and massage the gums with goldenseal tea (available at health food stores).

Myrrh (yes, one of the gifts brought by the wise men) is a shrub, and the gum from that shrub is an antiseptic and astringent used on bleeding or swollen gums to heal the infection that's causing the problem. Myrrh oil can be massaged directly on gums, or use myrrh powder on your soft-bristled toothbrush and gently brush your teeth at the gum line. Do it several times throughout the day.

In parts of Mexico, pyorrhea is treated by rubbing gums with the rattle from a rattlesnake. (We'd hate to think of how they do root canals.)

‡ PREPARING FOR DENTAL WORK

As soon as you know you're going to the dentist to have work done, start eating pineapple every day. Have fresh pineapple or a cup of canned pineapple in its own juice, and drink a cup of 100 percent pineapple juice. Continue the pineapple regime for a few days after the dental work is completed. The enzymes in pineapple should help reduce pain and discomfort. They can also help speed the healing process.

‡ TARTAR REMOVER

Mix equal parts of cream of tartar and salt. Brush your teeth and massage your gums with the mixture, then rinse very thoroughly.

‡ TEETH WHITENER

Burn a piece of toast. Really char it. (For some of us, that's part of our everyday routine.) Pulverize the charred bread, mix it with about ½ teaspoon of honey and brush your teeth with it. Rinse thoroughly; put on a pair of sunglasses; look in the mirror; and smile!

‡ DRY MOUTH

When it's time to make that all-important speech, or pop that critical question, you want to seem calm and sound confident. That's hard to do when your mouth is dry. When this happens, do not drink cold beverages. Doing so may help your dry mouth, but it will tighten up your already-tense throat. Also, stay away from drinks with milk or cream. They can create phlegm and more problems talking. Warm tea is your best bet. If there's none available, gently chew on your tongue. In less than twenty seconds, you'll manufacture all the saliva you'll need to end your dry mouth condition.

‡ CANKER SORES

Canker sores are painful, annoying, and can last for weeks. They are believed to be brought on by stress and have been linked to a deficiency of niacin. Take 50 to 100 mg of niacin daily. Don't be alarmed if you get a "flush" from the niacin, although it doesn't usually happen unless you take 125 mg or more. The redness, tingling, and itching do not last long and are completely harmless. Anyway, the daily dose of niacin may speed the healing process and also prevent a recurrence of the sores.

Get an ear of corn, discard the kernels, and burn a little piece of cob at a time. Apply the cob ashes to the canker sore three to five times a day. (Too bad this isn't a remedy for the toes. We'd have "cob on the corn.")

Several times throughout the day, keep a glob of black-strap molasses in your mouth on the canker sore. Molasses has extraordinary healing properties. Be sure to rinse thoroughly with water after using molasses.

According to psychic healer Edgar Cayce, castor oil is soothing and promotes healing of canker sores. Dab the sore with it each time the pain reminds you it's there.

‡ COLD SORES AND FEVER BLISTERS

Speed up the healing process of a cold sore by cutting a clove of garlic in half and rubbing it on the sore. Not pleasant, but effective.

Combine 1 tablespoon of apple cider vinegar with 3 tablespoons of honey (preferably raw honey) and dab the sore with the mixture in the morning, late afternoon, and at night.

Grind up a few walnuts and mix them with 1 teaspoon of cocoa butter. Apply this "nutty-butter" salve to the sore twice a day. The sore should be gone in three or four days.

Lysine may inhibit the growth of herpes viruses that cause cold sores and fever blisters. Take one L-lysine 500 mg tablet daily with dinner. See "Herpes" for more useful information.

This folk remedy came to us from several folks across the country. If they weren't embarrassed to tell it to us, we won't be embarrassed to tell it to you. Use earwax (your own, of course) on your cold sore or fever blister.

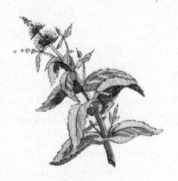

‡ BAD BREATH (HALITOSIS)

NOTE: It's important to find the cause of bad breath. Check for chronic sinusitis, or indigestion, and see a dentist.

While no one ever dies of bad breath, it sure can kill a relationship. Here are some refreshing remedies that are worth a try:

Suck on a piece of cinnamon bark to sweeten your breath. Cinnamon sticks come in jars or can be bought loose at some food specialty shops. They can also satisfy a craving for a sweet treat.

Bad breath is sometimes due to food particles decaying between one's teeth. If that's the case, use dental floss and brush after every meal.

Take a piece of 100 percent wool—preferably white and not dyed—put ½ teaspoon of raw honey on the fabric and massage your upper gums with it. Put another ½ teaspoon of raw honey on it and massage the lower gums. Did you say that sounds crazy? We can't argue with you there, but it's worth a try. Rinse thoroughly with water after using honey.

Use your toothbrush or a tongue scraper (available at pharmacies and health food stores) and scrape your tongue after breakfast and at bedtime.

Stock up on mint, rosemary, and fennel seeds (available at health food stores) and prepare an effective mouthwash for yourself. For a daily portion, use ⅓ teaspoon of each of the three dried herbs. Pour 1 cup of just-boiled water over the mint, rosemary, and fennel seeds, cover the cup, and let the mixture steep for ten minutes. Then strain it. At that point, it should be cool enough for you to rinse with. You might also want to swallow a little. It's wonderful for digestion, which may be causing the bad breath.

At bedtime, take a piece of myrrh the size of a pea and let it dissolve in your mouth. Since myrrh is an antiseptic and can destroy the germs that may cause the problem, hopefully you can say "bye-bye" to dragon breath.

It is believed that some cases of halitosis are caused by the stomach's faulty production of hydrochloric acid. It is also believed that niacin can regulate and even cure the problem. Taking niacin is quite an experience. Some people temporarily turn brick red all over from it. Joan gets horrible stomach pains for a few minutes, turns red all over, and itches. To prevent the niacin flush, take no more than 50 mg to 100 mg at any one time. Niacinamide offers the same benefits and none of the side effects.

When leaving an Indian restaurant, have you ever noticed a bowl filled with seeds that were there for the taking?

They are, most likely, anise. Suck on a few of those licorice-tasting seeds to sweeten your breath.

You may want to have a bowl of anise at your next dinner party.

‡ ONION AND GARLIC BREATH

Suck a lemon! It should make your onion or garlic breath disappear. Some people get better results when they add salt to the lemon, then suck it. (That's also a good remedy for getting rid of hiccups.)

CAUTION: Do not do this often. Do it only in an emergency social situation. The strongly acidic lemon juice is not good for tooth enamel.

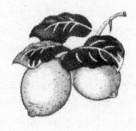

‡ Ulcers

A small percentage of people get ulcers from continual use of aspirin and other painkillers. If that doesn't apply to you, keep reading.

A recent incredible discovery was made about the *main* cause of ulcers. About 80 percent of all ulcers can be blamed on *Helicobacter pylori,* bacteria more commonly referred to as *H. pylori.* It is estimated that half of the American adult population has *H. pylori* present but dormant in their stomachs. Why do some people develop ulcers and others don't? Our commonsense guess is that emotional upsets, fatigue, nervous anxiety, chronic tension, and/or the inability to healthfully handle a high-pressure job or situation may devitalize the immune system, lowering one's resistance to the *H. pylori.*

If you're a member of this "fret set," we can suggest remedies for the ulcer, but you have to remedy the cause. Change jobs, meditate, look into self-help seminars, or do whatever is appropriate to transform your specific problem into something positive and happily manageable.

And now, we're asking you nicely: Please don't try any of these remedies without your doctor's blessing, okay?

According to a report in *Practical Gastroenterology,* "Aside from its failure to promote healing of gastric ulceration, the bland diet has other shortcomings: It is not palatable, and it is too high in fat and too low in roughage."

We also learned that milk may not be the cure-all we all thought it was. It may neutralize stomach acid at first, but because of its calcium content, gastrin is secreted. Gastrin is a hormone that encourages the release of more acid. Steer clear of milk.

A high-fiber diet is believed to be best for treatment of ulcers and prevention of relapses.

If your doctor approves, take 1 tablespoon of extravirgin, cold-pressed olive oil in the morning and 1 tablespoon in the evening. It may soothe and heal the mucous membrane that lines the stomach.

Barley and barley water are a soothing food and drink that help rebuild the stomach lining. Boil 2 ounces of pearled barley in 6 cups of water until there's about one half the water—3 cups—left in the pot. Strain. If necessary, add honey and lemon to taste. Drink it throughout the day. Eat the barley in soup, stew, or by itself.

Recent research has substantiated the effectiveness of cabbage juice, a century-old folk remedy, for relief of ulcers. While today's pressured lifestyle is quite conducive to ulcers, we, at least, have modern machinery to help with the cure: a juice extractor. Juice a cabbage and drink a cup of the juice right before each meal, then another cup before bedtime. Make sure the cabbage is fresh, not wilted. Also, drink the juice as soon as you prepare it. In other words, don't prepare it ahead of time and refrigerate it. It loses a lot of value that way. According to reports on test groups, pain, symptoms, and ulcers disappeared within two to three weeks after starting the cabbage juice regimen.

People ask, "Why cabbage?" We researched and found two reasons:

- Cabbage is rich in the nonessential amino acid glutamine. Glutamine helps the healthy stomach cells regenerate and stimulates the production of mucin, a mucoprotein that protects the stomach lining.
- Cabbage contains gefarnate, a substance that helps strengthen the stomach lining and replace cells. (It's also used in anti-ulcer drugs.)

Start juicing!

For the acute distress of ulcers (and gastritis), Dr. Ray C. Wunderlich, Jr., of the Wunderlich Center for Nutritional Medicine in St. Petersburg, Florida, recommends lecithin granules—1 heaping tablespoon as needed. Lecithin capsules will also suffice. Both are available at health food stores.

‡ Varicose Veins

You may be able to stop varicose veins from getting worse simply by the way you sit. *Never* sit with your legs crossed. In a relaxed way, keep your knees and ankles together and slightly slant your legs. It's graceful looking and doesn't add to the congestion that promotes varicose veins.

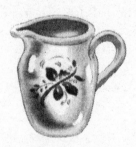

Folk medicine practitioners throughout Europe have been known to help shrink varicose veins by recommending the application of apple cider vinegar. Once in the morning and once in the evening, soak a cheesecloth bandage in the vinegar and wrap it around the affected area. Lie down, raise your legs, and relax that way for at least a half hour. This will benefit more than just your varicose vein condition. After each vinegar wrap session, drink 2 teaspoons of the vinegar in a cup of warm water. The practitioners tell us that by the end of one month, the veins shrink enough for there to be a noticeable difference.

In between the vinegar wraps, don't forget to sit properly (see the remedy above).

We'd be remiss not to tell you that if you're overweight, make a real effort to trim down. Your veins will be all the better for it.

Take vitamin C with bioflavonoids daily. Herbs may also be very helpful, particularly butcher's broom, horse chestnut, and hawthorn. You can find them in health food store. Follow the recommended dosage on the label.

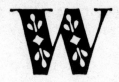

‡ Weight Control

This "weighty" subject is close to our heart, hips, thighs, midriff, stomach, and every other place we can pinch an inch or two or ten.

As hundreds of books and articles tell us, losing weight is hard; keeping it off is harder.

Most people go *on* a diet, living for the moment they can go *off* the diet.

The answer, then, is *not* to go on a diet. If you're not on a diet to begin with, you can't go off it, right?

We found some folk remedies that may help you lose weight without a temporary, I-can't-wait-to-go-off-it diet.

So, put some motivational reminders on your refrigerator—NOTHING STRETCHES SLACKS LIKE SNACKS! TO INDULGE IS TO BULGE! THOSE WHO LOVE RICH FOOD AND COOK IT, LOOK IT!—and start to practice "girth control."

NOTE: As for diet pills, they can be very helpful. Twice a day, we suggest you spill them on the floor and pick them up one at a time. It's great exercise, especially for the waistline.

‡ BASIC REDUCING PRINCIPLES

Try eating your larger meals early rather than late in the day. This gives your body lots of time to digest and burn off the calories. We've come across an appropriate saying: "Eat like a king in the morning, a prince at noon, and a pauper in the evening." While it's not always practical to have a four-course breakfast, you may want to eat a big lunch and a small dinner whenever you can.

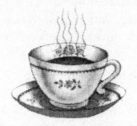

‡ ANCIENT SLIMMING HERBS

Each of the herbs we're going to mention here has several wonderful properties; the one they all have in common is the ability to help the user to be a loser . . . a weight loser.

Please know that these herbs do not give you license to start eating as though there's no tomorrow. They are tools that may help decrease the appetite and/or metabolize fat quickly, but they should be used in conjunction with a well-balanced eating plan.

You may want to taste each herb before deciding on the one to stick with for at least one month. The herbs are available in tea bags or loose at most health food stores.

To prepare, add 1 teaspoon of the dried, loose herb (or 1 tea bag) to a cup of just-boiled water. Cover it and let it steep for ten minutes. Strain and enjoy.

Drink 1 cup about a half hour before each meal and 1 cup at bedtime. It may take a month or two before you see results, especially if you hardly change your eating habits at all.

FENNEL SEEDS: The Greek name for fennel is *mara-thron,* from *mariano,* which means "to grow thin." Fennel is known to metabolize and throw off fatty substances through the urine. Fennel is rich in vitamin A and is wonderful for the eyes. It also aids digestion.

CLEAVERS: Like fennel seeds, cleavers is not known to lessen one's appetite, but to somehow accelerate fat metabolism. It's also a natural diuretic and can help relieve constipation. You may want to combine cleavers with fennel seeds as your daily drink.

RASPBERRY LEAVES: As well as having a reputation as a reducing aid, raspberry-leaf tea is said to help control diarrhea and nausea, help eliminate canker sores, and make pregnancy, delivery, and postdelivery easier for the mother-to-be.

YERBA MATÉ (Paraguay tea): We've heard that South American medical authorities who have studied yerba maté have concluded that this popular beverage can improve one's memory, nourish the smooth tissues of the intestines, increase respiratory power, help prevent infection, and is a tonic to the brain, nerves, and spine, as well as an appetite depressant and a digestive aid.

NOTE: Yerba maté contains caffeine (not as much as coffee). We were told that while it may act as a stimulant, it does not interfere with sleep.

HOREHOUND: This Old World herb is a diuretic and is used in cases of indigestion, colds, coughs, and asthma. It is also reported to be an effective aid for weight reduction.

SPIRULINA: This blue-green algae is an ancient Aztec food that's user-friendly. It's easily digestible, and is reported to enhance the immune system, help detoxify the body, and boost one's energy. Spirulina, taken daily, can help lift your spirits because of its high L-tryptophan content. As for helping you lose weight, take spirulina about twenty minutes before mealtime, and it may give you that full feeling, like you've already eaten a meal and hardly have room for more. Spirulina comes in several forms— powder, tablets, capsules, freeze-dried. Check it out at your health food store.

It most probably took you a while to reach your current weight. And it will take you a while to lose it. Be patient with yourself and give the herbs time to do their stuff. You can help the process along by eliminating or at least cutting down on foods with sugar, salt, and white flour.

Within a couple of months, you should be ready for the Nobelly prize!

‡ (NONHERBAL) SLIMMING SUGGESTIONS

We have a friend who's a light eater. As soon as it gets light, she eats. We told her about the grape juice remedy recommended by world-famous healer Edgar Cayce. Since starting this grape juice regimen, our friend's craving for desserts has almost disappeared, her eating patterns are gradually changing for the better, and she's fitting into clothes she hasn't worn in years.

Take 3 ounces of pure grape juice (no sugar, additives, or preservatives) mixed with 1 ounce of water a half hour before each meal and at bedtime. Drink the mixture slowly, taking from five to ten minutes to down each glass.

This Chinese acupressure technique is said to diminish one's appetite. Whenever you're feeling hungry, squeeze your earlobes for one minute. If you can stand the pressure, clamp clothespins on your lobes and leave them there for those sixty seconds.

We wonder if women who wear clip-on earrings are generally slimmer than women without them. Hmmmmm.

* * *

A woman we know dieted religiously. That means she wouldn't eat anything when she was in church. Out of control, desperate, and tired of all the fad diets, she came to us, looked in our "overweight" remedy file, and decided to follow the apple cider vinegar plan.

First thing in the morning, drink 2 teaspoons of apple cider vinegar in a glass of water. Drink the same mixture before lunch and dinner, making it three glasses of apple cider vinegar and water a day.

Within three months, the woman was no longer out of control or desperate. She felt that her days of binges were over and, thanks to the apple cider vinegar, she had the strength and willpower to stick to a well-balanced eating plan as the pounds slowly came off.

Lecithin is said to help break up and burn fatty deposits from stubborn bulges. It can also give you a full feeling after eating less than usual. The recommended daily dosage is 1 to 2 tablespoons of the lecithin granules.

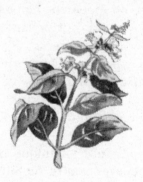

‡ THE DIET "BLUES"

Color therapist Carlton Wagner claims that blue food is unappetizing. Put a blue lightbulb in the refrigerator and a blue spotlight in your dining area. Wagner points out that restaurants know all about people's responses to the color blue when it comes to food. When serving food on blue plates, customers eat less, saving the restaurants money on their all-you-can-eat "Blue Plate" offers.

‡ LEG SLIMMING

Every night, rest your feet as high on a wall as is comfortable while you're lying on the floor or in bed. Stay that way for about an hour. At most, your legs will slim down. At least, it will be good for your circulation.

‡ Wilen Sisters' Sensational Six Superfoods

"Let food be your medicine." Hippocrates, the Greek physician known as the father of medicine, said those wise words sometime around 400 B.C. Those same words are being repeated today by many health professionals. After years of research, the scientific community recognizes the great value of food used for prevention and treatment of just about every ailment. Supplement companies certainly realize the healing power of food: they've been extracting and processing beneficial food substances for years, and packaging them in the form of pills, pearles, capsules, powders, tinctures, teas, creams, gels, and more.

With all due respect to Dr. Hippocrates, we would like to paraphrase his words of wisdom, to make them more appropriate for the information in this chapter: "Let food help prevent your need for medicine."

‡ EENEY, MEENEY, MINEY, MOTIVES

Our criteria for choosing the six superfoods was that each one had to be extremely health-giving in many ways, readily available, and affordable. Then we narrowed down our list by selecting foods that most people eat, or at least are familiar with, but might have no idea how very healthful they can be. That's how garlic, ginger, nuts, and yogurt made our list. Four down and two to go.

We then thought of having foods that need introducing. In other words, if not for reading about them here in these pages, you may not have known about them, and the big difference they can make in the way you eat and feel. That's how we decided on flaxseed and bee pollen to round out our Sensational Six Superfoods. Eating these superfoods regularly can go a long way toward alleviating conditions, preventing others, and helping you overcome the shortcomings of your gene pool.

‡ EXPAND YOUR HEALTHY HORIZONS

Read our Sensational Six Superfoods and consider working them into your daily diet. So as not to overwhelm yourself, add one or two new foods a week, replacing one or two less health-giving foods. Be creative. Experiment with different ways to prepare the foods; try different brands, different varieties. Approach it as a rewarding adventure. It will be.

Hearty appetite!

‡ #1. BEE POLLEN

The bee is awesome. Any engineer will tell you that, considering the size and shape of this creature, there is no way it should be able to fly. Honeybees are frequent flyers. Their flights from flower to flower are responsible for cross-pollination. In case you don't remember learning about it in school, here's a quick refresher course: Every flower produces pollen, which is the male reproductive element that is transferred by wind or insects (mostly bees) to fertilize the ovule of another flower. This tiny grain of pollen (it takes tens of millions to fill a spoon) has the power to produce the seed which can eventually become a flower, a bush, or a tree. The pollen that honeybees collect is, appropriately, called bee pollen.

‡ *Quality, Color, Taste, and What-For*

"The honeybee instinctively collects only the freshest and most potent pollen from what's available," says beekeeper James Hagemeyer, of Health from the Hive in Madisonville,

Tennessee. "There are numerous varieties of flowers in bloom at any given time, so the pollen collection varies with the season, resulting in all colors of pollen (from white to black and every color in between) with differing and distinctive tastes—some sweet and some bitter. The overall taste of most pollen is slightly bitter."

"Mr. Bee Pollen," as James Hagemeyer is known in the beekeeping community, tells everyone who will listen, "Although pollen is a food, not a drug, it shouldn't be eaten because it tastes good; it should be eaten because it's good for you!"

‡ Nature's Perfect Food

Referred to as the most complete food in nature, bee pollen has all of the necessary nutrients needed for human survival: at least eighteen of the twenty-two amino acids, more than a dozen vitamins—rich in B complex, A, C, D, and E, almost all known minerals, trace elements, eleven enzymes or co-enzymes, and fourteen beneficial fatty acids. Bee pollen contains the essence of every plant the bees visit, combined with the digestive enzymes from the bees.

It's 35 percent proteins, 55 percent carbohydrates, 2 percent fatty acids, and 3 percent vitamins and minerals. That leaves 5 percent unaccounted for. That 5 percent, which science has not yet been able to isolate and identify, may be what's alluded to in whispers as "the magic of the bee" that makes bee pollen so powerful.

‡ Pollen Power

According to naturopath Steve Schecter, more than forty research studies document the therapeutic efficacy and safety of bee pollen. Clinical tests show that orally ingested bee pollen particles are rapidly and easily absorbed; they pass directly from the stomach into the blood stream. Dr. Schecter's overview is that "bee pollen rejuvenates your body, stimulates organs and glands, enhances vitality, and brings about a longer life span."

Here are some specifics:

- *Bee pollen offers relief from allergies.* The pollen reduces the production of histamine, which can cause problems like hay fever. The pollen's protein can help the body build a natural defense against allergic reactions. To desensitize yourself, start taking bee pollen daily, a month or two before the start of hay-fever season.

  Do not confuse the pollen that the wind blows around, which is a *cause* of allergies, with bee pollen. The pollen collected by bees is heavier and stickier and even though it will rarely cause allergy symptoms, it is best to begin taking it in very small amounts. Start with just 1 or 2 granules the first day, and increase the amount daily until you reach your target dose (see "Forms and Dosage" on page 263. If, at any time, you have an allergic reaction like a rash, hives, wheezing, or swollen lips, take ¼ to ½ teaspoon of baking soda in water, and an antihistamine, and seek medical attention immediately. Needless to say, discontinue taking bee pollen.
- *Bee pollen is used by athletes to help increase their strength, endurance, energy, and speed.* Pollen is said to help the body recover from exercise, bringing the breathing and heart rate quickly back to normal.
- *Bee pollen can alleviate mental fatigue and improve alertness and concentration, helping you keep focused for longer periods of time.* It's reported that pollen improves the mental as well as the physical reactions of athletes.
- *Bee pollen has been known to promote fertility as well as sexual vitality.* Noel Johnson credits bee pollen as one of the reasons for writing his book, *A Dud at 70 . . . A Stud at 80!*
- *Noted Swedish dermatologist Dr. Lars-Erik Essen,*

who pioneered the use of bee products for skin conditions, said, "The skin becomes younger looking, less vulnerable to wrinkles, smoother, and healthier with the use of honeybee pollen."

- *Studies show that bee pollen, taken daily with a glass of water (about fifteen to thirty minutes before meals), can decrease food consumption by 15 to 20 percent.* Bee pollen is said to help correct a metabolic imbalance which may contribute to weight gain. The lecithin in pollen speeds up the burning of calories. It also may assist in the digestive process and the assimilation of nutrients.

- *Bee pollen protects against radiation's adverse effects, and helps strengthen the immune system.* We are all exposed to radiation (radioactive toxins) and chemical pollutants, which are known to cumulatively stress our immune system. According to Dr. Schecter's research, several nutrients in bee pollen, such as proteins, beneficial fats, vitamins B, C, D, E, and beta-carotene, calcium, magnesium, selenium, nucleic acids, lecithin, and cysteine, have been scientifically proven to strengthen immunity, counteract the effects of radiation and chemical toxins, and generate optimal health and vitality.

  Bee pollen significantly reduced the usual side effects of both radium and cobalt-60 radiotherapy in twenty-five women who had been treated for cancer. The women who took the pollen were considerably healthier, had stronger immune responses, and reported feeling an improved sense of well-being. The dosage of bee pollen prescribed for these women was approximately 2 teaspoons three times per day. (*Reminder:* This dosage should only be taken under the supervision of your health professional.)

‡ Forms and Dosage

Bee pollen comes in gelatin caps, tablets, and granules. We opt for the granules. We feel that the body absorbs the granules more efficiently and they're less processed. We take a teaspoon with water, before each meal. If we need a boost in energy, we take an extra teaspoon during the day.

Dr. Schecter reports that for preventive purposes, a common adult dosage of bee pollen granules is initially ⅛ to ¼ teaspoon once per day. The dosage is *gradually* increased to 1 to 2 teaspoons one to three times per day.

CAUTION: Adults suffering from allergies are best advised to start off with one to three granules daily, and then to gradually increase to higher doses, usually over a period of one month or more.

If you prefer to take bee pollen capsules for preventive purposes, the suggested amount is two 450 to 580 mg capsules three to four times daily. A short-term, therapeutic amount of bee pollen is about three times the preventive amount and should be taken only under the supervision of your health professional.

Be sure to buy bee pollen that comes from the U.S. Foreign pollens may be fumigated and baked.

Bee pollen should not be heated in any way. Keep it in the refrigerator. If, for economical reasons, you buy a large quantity, you can keep what you're not using in the freezer. James Hagemeyer said that viable bee pollen was found in five-thousand-year-old Egyptian tombs. If it kept that long in tombs, it should keep at least a thousand years in the freezer!

‡ Bee Pollen for Animals

Have you noticed that dogs seem to be suffering from the same health challenges as humans? According to Janet Lipa, breeder of golden retrievers and owner of Golden Tails, a holistic food company for animals, overvaccinating pets, particularly purebred dogs, may be responsible for the animals' health problems. Those annual inoculations may cause the buildup of toxins in the liver, compromising the immune system and making the animal more susceptible to illness.

Bee pollen can help boost the immune system, and help your pet get rid of allergies—runny eyes, itchy skin.

For a thousand-pound horse, mix 1 heaping tablespoon of bee pollen in the A.M. feeding, and repeat in the P.M. feeding. First check with your vet.

For other animals, use ⅛ teaspoon per 15 pounds of body weight. Mix the bee pollen in with the food in the morning and repeat in the afternoon feeding. Allow thirty to sixty days to see results. You may want to check with your vet first.

‡ *Make a Beeline* . . .

Your local beekeeper or health food store should have bee pollen. The "Sources" chapter in this book can also point you in the right direction for you to bee all that you can bee.

‡ #2. FLAX—SEEDS AND OIL

People have been eating flaxseed for thousands of years. In the south—that is, southern Mesopotamia, c. 5200–4000 B.C.—records show that irrigation was used to grow flax. The Babylonians cultivated flaxseed as early as 3000 B.C., and, wouldn't you know, Hippocrates used flaxseed for the relief of intestinal discomfort. "Take two tablespoons of flaxseed and call me in the morning."

Dr. Stephan Cunnane, professor of nutritional sciences at the University of Toronto, said, "Flaxseed will be the nutraceutical food of the twenty-first century because of its multiple health benefits." That makes sense to us, and here's why:

‡ *What's So Great about Flax*

Flax oil, processed from flaxseed, contains the highest concentration of *essential* omega-3 of any other source on the planet. A deficiency of omega-3 has been positively correlated with over sixty illnesses, including: arthritis, atherosclerosis, cancer, diabetes, hypertension (high blood pressure), immune disorders, menopausal discomfort, and stroke. And so, adding omega-3 supplementation to your daily diet may go a long way in helping to prevent, improve, or reverse those unhealthy conditions.

Flaxseed contains phytonutrients called lignans. Lignans are reported to have the following attributes: antitumor properties; estrogen-mimicking effect without risks associated with estrogen therapy; powerful antioxidant capabilities; antiviral properties; antibacterial properties; and antifungal properties. Studies suggest that lignans may help prevent many health problems, including breast and colon cancer, and can help lower cholesterol, regulate women's menstrual cycles, and reduce or eliminate menopausal symptoms.

‡ *Flax—Seeds and/or Oil—and Dosage*

If you're thinking that flaxseed, in some form, should be part of your daily diet, we think it's a wise decision. To help you decide which form(s) to take, you should know: Flaxseeds have hard outer shells. You can eat them *after* you've soaked a few tablespoons of the seeds overnight. Or, the most popular way to eat flaxseeds is to grind them in a spice or coffee grinder. Then sprinkle a tablespoon of the ground meal on your cereal, or add it to a smoothie, or mix it into a portion of fat-free yogurt or fat-free cottage cheese. When baking, you can replace a few tablespoons of your regular flour with flax flour.

To make sure we get our daily dose of the omega-3 oils and lignans, we ourselves find it most convenient to take flax oil. We were advised to start with 2 tablespoons a day—one in the morning, and one either in the afternoon or evening. Then, after a couple of months, regulate the daily dosage to a tablespoon of flax oil per every hundred pounds of body weight.

We add the flax oil to a smoothie—it doesn't change the taste of the smoothie, it just keeps it from getting very aerated, which is a good thing—or we mix flax oil in fat-free yogurt, along with a minced clove of garlic. It's good! We also use flax oil in a homemade salad dressing. There are lots of recipes using flax oil. (See the "Recommended Reading" chapter for a flax oil cookbook.)

When we first started looking for flax oil, we went to the refrigerated section of our local health food store and found Barlean's Flax Oil. (See "Natural Foods and More" in the "Sources" chapter.) It had all of the qualities we were looking for, including and especially "Lignan Rich." (Typically, lignans, the important phytoestrogens that may help prevent cancer, are not present in appreciable amounts in most flaxseed oils—Barlean's is one of the exceptions.) Also, due to flaxseed oil's limited shelf life—it's an oil that can become rancid and should be kept refrigerated—we checked the "pressing date" and the "best before date," making sure they didn't exceed a four-month span.

‡ Your Life in the Balance

For those of you who want more of the whole picture of essential fatty acids in our body, Jade Beutler, a licensed health care practitioner and author of *Flax for Life*, agreed to share some information with us.

Health, life and longevity critically rely on a delicate balance of two *essential* nutrients. The imbalance of these two vital nutrients is credited as possibly the leading cause of death and disability in America today.

Both Omega-3, found abundantly in flax oil, and Omega-6, found in a plethora of processed oils—including corn, safflower and sunflower—have been deemed as *essential* nutrients by the World Health Organization. As *essential* nutrients, we must get these *essential* fatty acids (EFAs) directly in the foods we eat, or via nutritional supplementation. The body cannot manufacture them from other nutrients.

According to Artemis Simopoulos, M.D., President of the Center of Genetics, Nutrition and Health, "Throughout human history, Omega-3 and Omega-6 fatty acids have been ingested in near-perfect proportion. That is to say, roughly a 50/50 concentration. For millions of years, the equal ingestion of these two EFA's has created a delicate check-and-balance system within the body, and in control of, literally, thousands of metabolic functions. That means everything including immune function, cellular communication, insulin sensitivity, and inflammatory response hormone and steroid production. It is impossible for optimal health to be attained with a *tissue* imbalance of Omega-3 to Omega-6 fatty acids.

‡ *Fooling Mother Nature?*
"Within the last 100 years, coinciding with the industrial revolution, has come the processing of seeds that are dominant in Omega-6 oils," explains Beutler.

These oils, once ingested moderately in the diet, are now ingested disproportionately as vegetable oil and in fried and processed foods that contain them.

Removing Omega-3 fatty acids from the food chain has compounded the problem. Food manufacturers were quick to find out that Omega-3 fatty acids greatly diminished the desired shelf life of 1 to 2 years. Therefore Omega-3's are either removed from the food, or avoided entirely.

Modern methods of animal husbandry call on the predominant use of Omega-6 dominant seeds and oils to *fatten* the livestock up for slaughter. As a result, animal meats that once provided a concentrated source of Omega-3 are now nearly completely devoid of it, while teeming with Omega-6.

‡ Consequences and Conclusions

Beutler's research has led him to the realization that, "The mass ingestion of Omega-6 at the expense of Omega-3 has created a drastic shift in human biophysiology." The Japanese, after reviewing more than five hundred studies on the subject, concluded: "The evidence indicates that increased dietary linoleic acid (Omega-6) and relative Omega-3 deficiency are major risk factors for western-type cancers, cardiovascular and cerebrovascular diseases, and also for allergic hyper-reactivity. We also raise the possibility that a relative Omega-3 deficiency may be affecting the behavioral patterns of a proportion of the young generations in industrialized countries."

‡ Getting Back to Balance

According to Simopoulos, it would take the human body one million years to adapt to the drastic shift in ingestion of omega-3 to omega-6 fatty acids that has occurred in only the last hundred years. "The implication is clear," says Beutler. "And so is the solution. We must consciously shift the Omega-3/Omega-6 balance by supplementing our diet with Omega-3 to avert otherwise certain degenerative disease."

As mentioned before, "Flax oil contains the highest concentration of *essential* omega-3 of any other source on the planet."

‡ #3. GARLIC

When it comes to garlic, we wrote the book. We *really* did. It's appropriately called, *Garlic—Nature's Super Healer*

(Prentice Hall). In the book, we talk about how you can use the healing power of garlic for more than ninety ailments. If you check out the index in this book, you'll see many uses for the "stinking rose."

Garlic is a natural antibiotic with antiviral, antifungal, anticoagulant, and antiseptic properties. It can act as an expectorant and decongestant, antioxidant, germicide, anti-inflammatory agent, diuretic, sedative, and it is believed to contain cancer-preventive chemicals. It's also said to be an aphrodisiac, but you must find a partner who also eats garlic.

‡ Why the Smell

Once a garlic clove is bruised in any way (cut, crushed, mashed, pressed, diced, sliced, minced), through a highly complex conversion process, *allicin* is formed and spontaneously decomposes into a group of odoriferous compounds which provide much of garlic's medicinal punch.

‡ How to Eat Raw Garlic

Using garlic in cooking is fine, but when garlic is heated, it loses some of its health-giving power. Garlic gurus agree that raw garlic does the most good as an antibiotic and as preventive medicine.

Eating raw garlic on an empty stomach may cause burning, irritation, and discomfort. Don't do it!

The most delicious and soothing way to eat raw garlic is to mix a minced clove into a dollop of plain, nonfat yogurt or fat-free cottage cheese. After reading the information on flax oil, you may also want to mix in a tablespoon of flax oil, making it an extremely healthy snack. Anna Maria Clement, co-director of Hippocrates Health Institute in West Palm Beach, Florida, recommends a variation of that. She says to put a tablespoon of flaxseed in a glass of water and leave it overnight. In the morning, the flaxseed in water will be of a viscous consistency. Stir it and drink it. It will protect your stomach so that you can eat a clove or two of raw garlic.

Brian Clement of Hippocrates says to take a big bite of apple (organic, of course) and chew it thoroughly, letting the apple's pectin get around your mouth before swallowing. Then pop a raw garlic clove. There shouldn't be any burning, thanks to the enzymes and pectin in the apple.

Minced garlic in apple sauce is also a tasty, painless way to eat raw garlic. Incidentally, if you don't chew the finely minced garlic, you will not have garlic breath.

Also, sprinkle raw, minced garlic on a salad, or prepare dressing with it.

‡ Shopping for Garlic

Buy bulbs that are sold loose rather than packaged so that you can see and feel them.

The papery, outer skin should be taut and unbroken.

Beware of sprouting green shoots, discoloration, mold, rot (feel for soft spots), or shriveling. When garlic gets old, it dries out, its flavor dissipates, and it becomes bitter.

Look for garlic bulbs that are plump, solid, and heavy for their size.

A bulb has anywhere from eight to forty cloves. Average is about fifteen cloves. Look for bulbs with large cloves so you can cut down on peeling time.

‡ Storing Garlic

Store garlic bulbs away from any heat source like a stove or the sun. A cool, dry, dark place is ideal, and in an open container, a crock with ventilation holes, or a net bag that allows air to circulate around them.

Do not freeze uncooked garlic. Its consistency will break down and it will have an awful, ungarlicky smell.

Homemade preparations containing garlic-in-oil must be

refrigerated. Put a date on the label. *Do not* keep it longer than two weeks! Rancid oil can be dangerous.

‡ *Garlic Supplements*

Commercial supplements should not be chosen by impressive advertising campaigns, and high-priced pills do not mean they're better.

"Basically, it's a consumer-beware market for garlic supplements," says Elizabeth Somer, M.A., R.D. "Some garlic products have 33 times more of certain compounds than other garlic products. Unless the label lists specific amounts (per capsule or tablet) of active ingredients such as allicin, S-allyl-cysteine, ajoene, dialyl sulfides, or at least total sulfur content, then assume the product is 'condiment grade' and no better or worse than garlic powder seasoning, just a lot more expensive." We think it's important that the label says "allicin" or "allicin potential" and lists one or more of the other active ingredients mentioned above.

Varro E. Tyler, professor of pharmacognosy (drugs from natural sources) at Purdue University, told us that *enteric-coated* garlic supplements are recommended for maximum absorption of allicin. A supplement that is enteric-coated resists the effects of stomach acid and allows the intestinal enzymes to dissolve it so that the full benefit of the supplement is obtained. Check labels for the words "enteric-coated" as well as "allicin."

CAUTION: Too much raw garlic can cause headaches, diarrhea, gas, fever, and in extreme cases, gastric bleeding. This garlic is strong stuff! Do not overdo it.

WARNING: Do not eat garlic or take garlic supplements if you have a bleeding disorder, or ulcers, or are taking anticoagulants.

WISE SUGGESTION: If you are taking any kind of medication, check with your health professional before starting any self-help treatment.

‡ #4. GINGER: AN ANCIENT REMEDY PERFECT FOR TODAY

What are friends for? To share their expertise with you and your readers—that is, if you're lucky enough to be friends with Paul Schulick, research herbalist, author (see "Recommended Reading") and one of the world's leading authorities on one of the "Sensational Six Superfoods." Here is Paul Schulick's important input on ginger.

"Doctor," said the imaginary patient, "I have a host of serious problems." The doctor listened carefully and compassionately (remember, this is make-believe) as the patient recounted the ailments. "Doctor, I think I have parasites, and they make me nauseated all the time. In addition, my family has a history of colon cancer, and I have some blood in my stool. And I suppose I could handle that, but I feel feverish, and my joints constantly ache. I started out this year at five feet, seven inches, and I think I must be shrinking. Also, my cholesterol is elevated, and I was taking aspirin to avoid blood clotting, but it tore my stomach up. I think I now have ulcers! Doctor, what should I take? And don't prescribe too much, because my memory is not what it used to be."

The doctor listened to this patient and then told him about the medicinal power of one herb that might just be the answer for all the problems. The doctor told the story of *Zingiber officinale,* commonly known as "ginger." This common herb, really a rhizome, has some profound and scientifically well-documented healing properties. The doctor told the patient to listen, but not to worry about memorizing the features:

1. Antiparasitic (against schistosoma mansoni, anisakis, dirofilaria immitis).
2. Antibacterial and antiviral (against staph, E. coli, salmonella, and strep).

3. Anti-emetic (for relief from nausea)—more effective than prescription drug metoclopramide.

4. Antimutagenic (cancer preventative)—against COX-2 related cancers (colon, pancreas, skin, esophageal), leukemia, and multiple tumor growth factors.

5. Balances and modulates inflammatory hormones associated with arthritis.

6. Balances and modulates the enzyme 5-lipoxygenase, which is associated with prostate and breast cancers, bone resorption (osteoporosis), and conditions of inflammation. (There are twenty-two known 5-lipoxygenase inhibitors.)

7. Inhibits the COX-2 enzyme associated with brain inflammation and with the neuronal death in Alzheimer's disease. (There are three known COX-2 inhibitors: melatonin, kaempferol, and curcumin.)

8. Powerful antioxidant, enhances the potency of other antioxidants. Contains at least twelve known anti-aging constituents that inactivate free radicals.

9. Wound healing and anti-ulcerative. More wound healing compounds than any other botanical.

10. Aphrodisiac.

11. Antihistaminic.

12. Powerful digestive enzyme—ginger has *180 times* the protein-digesting power of papaya.

13. Supports the growth of beneficial bacteria in our colon, specifically *Lactobacillus plantarum*, by a factor of five.

14. Modulates thromboxane, the hormone responsible for blood platelet aggregation and blood clotting, thus protecting against heart attack and stroke. More effective in this respect than garlic.

15. Reverses the inflammation associated with rheumatoid arthritis more effectively than prescription drugs, according to international medical research.

16. Increases bile secretion for better fat metabolism.
17. Lowers serum cholesterol.
18. Contains eleven sedative compounds, more than any other spice.

The patient listened with astonishment. "Do you mean to tell me that one drug can do all that?" The doctor replied, "No, I am not talking about a drug. Remember, I am that rare M.D. who is open to the phytomedicinal power of healing botanicals. I am talking about 'ginger,' which is absolutely NOT a drug. A drug has one synthetic molecule, and ginger has at least 477 natural compounds, all working together to promote safe and balanced healing."

This conversation may never have occurred in any M.D.'s office that you have visited, but people are starting to talk about ginger. It is long overdue. For thousands of years ginger has been known in Ayurvedic medicine as *vishwabhesaj,* the Universal Medicine. It is said that Confucius considered no meal complete without ginger, it was the Alka-Seltzer of the Roman Empire, and it was so valuable to Arab traders that purchasers were told that ginger came from the mythical kingdom of Xanadu so as to hide its true origins. And to top it all off, its invigorating taste has stimulated palates and calmed stomachs for thousands of years, and high-quality ginger remains a prized commodity.

There are several ways to enjoy the benefits of ginger. Fresh ginger is delightful, but it is important to use organic ginger, because *conventional* (better described as *chemically grown*) ginger is often heavily fumigated. It can be purchased dried and ground, which is a fine way to obtain the intestinal and protein-digesting benefits of the whole-fiber herb. Extracts are available of the fresh ginger juice, which can be used to make hot or cold teas or ginger ales. Ginger also *potentiates* or increases the power of other herbs, so it is valuable to use with green tea, echinacea, ginseng, and kava. Most recently, a new extract of ginger called a "Supercritical Extract" has become available, which allows you to take a powerful and pure concentrate (up to 250 to 1) of the healing, pungent compounds. But most important, organic ginger belongs in your daily life, for it is simply one of the finest (if not the finest) daily tonics available from the botanical world.

‡ #5. NUTS

Nuts! For years neither of us ate nuts. We love nuts but didn't eat them because they're so high in fat. And then, one day in the mid-1990s, we read an article extolling the health-giving properties of nuts, fat and all. What a wonderful surprise! The article reported the findings of the Loma Linda University, School of Public Health, Nutrition Department's research team, headed by Joan Sabaté, M.D., Ph.D., and associate professor of nutrition and epidemiology. We immediately called the university, and got another surprise. Dr. Joan Sabaté is a *man*—"Joan" being a man's name in Spain and Portugal—and one who was willing to share his research.

‡ *Results of Studies*

Starting in the mid-1970s, a team of epidemiologists at Loma Linda followed the eating habits of more than twenty-five thousand Seventh Day Adventists. At the end of ten years, the researchers found that there was only one common food linked to good health: nuts. Dr. Sabaté said, "The results couldn't have been more striking. People who ate nuts often—five or more times a week—were half as likely to have a heart attack or die of heart disease as people who rarely or never ate them. Eating nuts just one to four times a week cuts the heart risk by 25 percent." The doctor said it didn't matter if people were slim or fat, young or old, active or sedentary.

Dr. Sabaté conducted his own study with two groups of people. Both groups ate a typical American Heart Association cholesterol-lowering diet—the kind that doctors would recommend. In addition to the food allowed on the diet, one group had 2 to 3 ounces of walnuts daily and the other group had no walnuts. The cholesterol levels went down in both groups, but more so among the walnut eaters. Their blood cholesterol levels dropped twenty-two points in a few weeks.

Many studies of the effects of nuts have been done—an almond study in the Health Research and Studies Center in Los Altos, California, a walnut study at the University of California at San Francisco, a Harvard School of Public Health study involving 86,000 nurses, a Harvard Physicians Health study with 22,000 doctors, another study with 31,000 vegetarians, and still another with 40,000 postmenopausal women—and the results all point to the same conclusion: Nuts are a health-giving superfood!

‡ *Health Benefits—in a Nutshell*

All nuts contain flavonoids, which are potent antioxidants that help protect against cancer and heart disease.

Nuts are one of the best vegetable sources of vitamin E. They also have B vitamins—thiamine, niacin, folic acid, and riboflavin. Most nuts are rich in potassium needed to help regulate blood pressure and heart rate. Nuts are also a source for the fatigue and stress-fighting minerals iron, magnesium, and zinc. (Almonds and pecans are particularly rich in magnesium; cashews and pecans are rich in zinc.)

Nuts are packed with the antioxidants selenium and copper. (Brazil nuts are particularly rich in selenium; cashews, filberts, and walnuts are rich in copper.) In the sixteenth and seventeenth centuries, it was thought that various foods helped heal the body parts that they resembled. And so, our ancestors believed that walnuts helped the head and brain. They may have been right. Walnuts are a good source of copper, an essential mineral for maintenance of the nervous system *and* brain activity!

While most nuts have some calcium, almonds have more than any other nut; Brazil nuts and filberts also have substantial amounts of calcium.

An ounce of nuts gives you as much fiber as two slices of whole wheat bread. Almonds have the highest dietary fiber content of any nut.

Nut protein is loaded with the amino acid arginine, known to protect arteries from injury and to stop blood clots from forming.

Nuts contain phytochemicals (plant sterols or phytosterols which help lower cholesterol and are thought to protect against colon cancer); antioxidants (which protect against heart disease and cancer); saponins (which help lower cholesterol and also show evidence of having anti-cancer properties); and phytic acid or phytate (which has been found to be protective against colon cancer).

‡ *Nutty Facts (In Case You're on a TV Game Show)*
- The oldest food tree known to humankind is the walnut tree. It dates back to 7000 B.C.
- The nut with the highest fat content (over 70 percent) is the pecan.
- Cashew shells are thick, leathery, and have a blackish-brown oil that causes the skin to blister in a way similar to poison ivy.
- You may know that filberts are also called hazelnuts, but do you know another name for them? Cobnuts.
- Brazil nuts have the hardest shell of all nuts. Before cracking them, or any hard-shell nut, put them in the freezer for six hours. The deep-freeze makes the shells crack much easier.

- Peanuts are really legumes, which are nutritionally similar enough to nuts to include them as part of your health-giving food regimen.
- Nuts in their shells stay fresh twice as long as shelled nuts. If kept in a cool, dry place, raw, unshelled nuts can keep for six months to a year. But why would you want to keep them that long? Eat 'em!

‡ *Dosage*

Nuts have helped us change the way we think of fats. We now know that there are good fats, the unsaturated fats, the kind found in flaxseed, cold-water fish, avocado, and, of course, in nuts.

Dr. Joan Sabaté told us that 1 to 2 ounces of either almonds, cashews, pistachios, walnuts, or even peanuts five times a week is a heart-healthy amount to eat.

Be sure the nuts are raw. Organically grown is best. Stay away from the dyed red (how and why did *that* get started?) and salted pistachios. If you want peanut butter, the best is the kind you grind yourself at a health food store. Don't even think about commercial peanut butter with all the additives and preservatives.

For optimum health, don't just add nuts to your diet. Let nuts take the place of saturated, unhealthy fat. Cut back on meat and cheese and french-fried potatoes. Keep working your way toward a predominantly plant-based diet.

Gene Spiller, Ph.D. and author of *Healthy Nuts* (see the "Recommended Reading" chapter), thinks that nuts are so nutrient rich that they quell hunger pangs. It's possible that by eating nuts, you won't want to eat as much of everything else.

A nutritionist/spokesperson for Weight Watchers said that the problem with nuts is that once you start . . . Too much of a good thing is no longer a good thing. Don't go nuts!

‡ #6. YOGURT

In Egypt it's called *benraid*. The Armenians call it *may-zoom*. The Persian word is *kast*. In Turkey it's known as *yo-gurut*, from which our word *yogurt* is derived.

Although people have been making and eating yogurt for more than four thousand years, it took the research of No-bel Prize–winning scientist Ilya Metchnikoff in the beginning of the twentieth century to stir up European interest in yo-gurt, which eventually made its way to America in about 1940. In the 1950s, its reputation as a healthy, nutritional food started to spread across the country. Today yogurt production is a major industry.

‡ The Culture Club

Yogurt is most often made with the milk of cows. It can also be made with milk from goats, sheep, and buffalo, or with soymilk. Once the milk is pasteurized, many com-mercial yogurt producers enrich it with powdered milk. So when ads say that the yogurt has more protein and calcium than milk, it's true.

To meet the legal definition of *yogurt*, it is required that two cultures be added. These cultures break down the lac-tose (milk sugar), producing lactic acid and giving yogurt its unique taste. The live, active cultures are primarily what make yogurt a health-giving superfood.

‡ Health Benefits

Thanks to the live cultures, yogurt is a soothing and easily digested food, even for people who are lactose intolerant. In fact, yogurt helps digestion and, as a result, may clear up bad breath caused by stomach acid imbalances.

Yogurt is not only a good source of calcium, but the lac-tose helps improve calcium absorption. People at risk for osteoporosis should consider including a portion in their daily diet.

Yogurt contains B_{12}, riboflavin, potassium, magnesium,

and zinc. It's also a wonderful source of protein. The U.S. Department of Agriculture includes yogurt as a meat alternative in school lunches.

Studies show that eating a daily 8-ounce serving of yogurt with active bacterial cultures restores and maintains a healthy bacterial environment that can help prevent both bladder infections and vaginal yeast infections.

Antibiotics destroy friendly bacteria. A good way to replace them? Yogurt! After a bout of diarrhea, yogurt can help reestablish bacterial balance. Studies show that yogurt can decrease the duration of an attack of diarrhea in infants and children.

Studies also indicate that *Lactobacillus acidophilus* helps lower cholesterol by interfering with cholesterol reabsorption in the intestine.

All of the live cultures of bacteria in yogurt can enhance immunity, kill off certain unwanted strains of unhealthy bacteria, and increase production of antibodies (the natural killers of disease organisms) in your blood.

What's great is that those beneficial bacteria stay in your system and continue to help long after the yogurt is gone.

‡ *What to Look For*

First and foremost, whether you want regular, low-fat, or fat-free yogurt, be sure that the label says it contains "live" or "active" cultures. Most yogurt companies list their specific live cultures. Look for and expect to find at least one, maybe two or three (more is better), of the following friendly and helpful bacteria:

> Lactobacillus acidophilus
> Lactobacillus bulgaricus
> Lactobacillus casei
> Lactobacillus reuteri
> Streptococcus thermophilus
> Bifidobacteria

If fruit is mixed through yogurt, there's not much chance of there being live or active cultures. Buy plain yogurt and add a banana, berries, peaches, or pineapple—one of your five daily cancer-risk-reducing servings of fresh fruit. It also tastes great with a little honey mixed in.

See what other ingredients are listed on the label. You do *not* want additives and artificial sweeteners.

Before buying yogurt, check the expiration date and be sure it has not exceeded that date, or even come close.

If you really get into yogurt, you may want to try making your own. Kits are available in some health food stores. You'll need yogurt as a starter to make more yogurt. That's one way of testing the store-bought product for live cultures. If the cultures are alive and well, they will help produce more yogurt.

Sorry, but none of the health benefits apply to frozen yogurt. *Freezing* destroys the good stuff. There is also the unwanted presence of sugar or aspartame and lots more ingredients on the less-than-healthy list.

‡ *The Last Word on Yogurt*

In several ancient Middle Eastern languages, the word for *yogurt* was synonymous with *life*.

Remedies in a Class by Themselves

‡ **KISS-KISS**

There is a Kiel Osculatory Research Center in Germany, where scientists are studying the act of kissing. One of their findings is that the morning "Good-bye, dear," kiss is the most important one of the day. It helps start the day with a positive attitude that leads to better work performance and an easier time coping with stress. According to the researchers, that morning send-off kiss on a daily basis can add up to earning more money and living a longer, healthier life.

Hey, what about us single people? I don't know about you, but I'm going to make a deal with my doorman.

‡ **LUNG POWER**

This remedy requires an investment of some money and time. Increase your lung power and breath control by taking up a musical instrument—the harmonica (mouth organ). It's fun! You can buy a "Marine Band" by Hohner. That's a good beginner's harmonica and it's inexpensive. Hohner also publishes books that teach you to play the harmonica while you strengthen your lungs. Who knows—it may start you on a whole new career.

Playing the harmonica has even been known to alleviate symptoms of emphysema.

‡ YAWNING

Do not stifle a yawn. Yawning restores the equilibrium between the air pressure in the middle ear and that of the outside atmosphere, giving you a feeling of relief. And you thought you were just bored.

‡ IMMUNE SYSTEM STRENGTHENER

We've all heard that "confession is good for the soul." According to Dr. James W. Pennebaker, professor of psychology at the University of Texas and author of *Opening Up: The Healing Power of Expressing Emotions* (Guilford Press), "When we inhibit feelings and thoughts, our breathing and heart beat speed up, putting an extra strain on our autonomic nervous system." By writing about the stresses in your life, you release pent-up emotions, freeing the immune system to do its real job, that of guarding the body against unwanted invaders. After following Dr. P's formula exactly as directed, you should feel lighter, happier, and may experience better health during the next six months than you have during the last six months.

Dr. Pennebaker's Process

1) Find a quiet place where you can be alone for twenty minutes.
2) Write down a confession of what's bothering you. Be as specific as you can.
3) Don't worry about spelling or grammar. Just write continuously for the entire twenty minutes.
4) Keep going, even if it feels awkward. Letting go takes practice. If you reach a mental block, repeat your words.
5) After four days of writing, you should be ready to throw the paper away and enjoy your newly recharged immune system.

6) Feel free to repeat this exercise anytime something stressful comes up. Regular release will keep your immune system strong.

‡ NAPPING

It is said that a nap during the day can do wonders for balancing emotions and attitudes and, in general, harmonizing one's system without interference from the conscious mind.

Presidents Truman, Kennedy, and Johnson were well-known nappers. Add to that prestigious list of productive people who caught some shut-eye on a daily basis, Edison, Churchill, and, appropriately, *Nap*oleon.

‡ PRACTICE PREVENTIVE MEDICINE: LAUGH!

Writer and magazine editor Norman Cousins used laughter as a medicine to help overcome his doctor-diagnosed "incurable" disease.

According to Cousins, who referred to laughter as "inner jogging," there's scientific proof that it oxygenates the blood, improves respiration, stimulates the body's immune system, and helps release substances described as "the body's anesthesia and a relaxant that helps human beings to sustain pain."

Log on to a search engine, ask for "jokes" or "humor," and laugh it up!

‡ HAVE A GOOD CRY

Emotional tears have a higher protein content than onion-produced tears. A researcher at the St. Paul–Ramsey Medical Center accounts for that difference as nature's way of releasing chemical substances (the protein) created during an emotional or stressful situation. In turn, the release of those chemical substances allows the negative feelings to flow out, letting a sense of well-being return.

According to Dr. Margaret Crepeau of Marquette University, people who suppress tears are more vulnerable to disease. In fact, suppressing any kind of feeling seems to take its toll on one's system. Face your feelings and let 'em out!

‡ CALCIUM CONCERN

The body is robbed of calcium when there is a high consumption of caffeine, colas, and other soft drinks. Also, calcium absorption is compromised in people who smoke, take antacids that are high in aluminum, or are on a low-sodium diet and/or on a high-protein diet. We should all—particularly women—eat foods rich in calcium: canned sardines, canned salmon, soybean products including tofu, dark green leafy vegetables, asparagus, blackstrap molasses, sunflower seeds, sesame seeds, walnuts, almonds, peanuts, dried beans, corn tortillas, and dairy products.

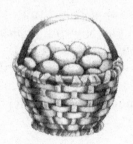

‡ CHASING THE BLUES AWAY

To lighten a heavy heart, drink saffron tea and/or thyme tea, sweetened with honey. (Incidentally, "thyme" was originally called "wild time" because it was thought to be an aphrodisiac.)

Sniffing citrus essential oils each hour you're awake may help you get out of a funk. You can buy lemon or orange oil at a health food store. DO NOT take the essential oils internally. If you have a citrus fruit in your kitchen, you can use a cardboard cutter to carefully make slits in the peel and squeeze it so that the volatile oil seeps out. Then take a whiff hourly.

If you're mildly depressed and don't want to be, simply change your physiology and your emotions will follow suit. In other words, do the physical things you do when you're happy and you'll get happy. Smile! Laugh! Jump up and down! Sing! Dance! Get dressed up!

If you're not willing to go along with this suggestion, then you're not willing to let go of your depression. There's nothing wrong with staying in a funk as long as you understand that it is your choice.

‡ LONGEVITY

In ancient Babylonian, Egyptian, Persian, and Chinese texts, one folk food is considered to be the secret ambrosia of youth; the formula for glowing health; the magic key to longevity. This folk food is bee pollen.

Take 1 tablespoon of bee pollen every day and when you're a healthy hundred-year-old who looks seventy, you'll know it works. Read all about bee pollen in the "Sensational Six Superfoods" chapter.

‡ GIVE HEALING ORDERS

A Johns Hopkins Hospital survey concluded that three out of four ailments stemmed from emotional factors. It makes sense. Crises in our lives cause emotional reactions which cause biochemical changes that disrupt the body's harmony, weaken immunity, and upset hormone production.

We do it to ourselves; we can undo it!

Relax every part of your body (follow the visualization exercise in the "Nervous Tension, Anxiety, and Stress" chapter). Once you're completely relaxed, order your body to heal itself. Actually give your body commands out loud. Be direct, clear, and positive. Picture your specific problem. (There's no right or wrong; it's all up to your own imagination.) Once you have a clear picture of your problem, see it healing. Envision pain flying out of your pores; picture the condition breaking up and disintegrating. Say and see whatever seems appropriate for your particular case.

End this daily session by looking in the mirror and repeating a dozen times, "Wellness is mine," AND MEAN IT!

Facts and Food for Thought

‡ GOOD HEALTH ITALIAN STYLE

It's unusual to find on-in-years Italians with asthma, tuberculosis, or gallbladder trouble, thanks to the garlic and olive oil they use in two out of their three daily meals.

‡ KNUCKLE CRACKING

According to an informal study conducted at UCLA, the gruesome habit of knuckle cracking does not lead to arthritic problems later on . . . just a lot of unpleasantness now: "Will you stop that? You're getting on my nerves. I can't take that cracking anymore!"

‡ CRADLING BABY

The Talmud (ancient Hebrew writings) suggests that a woman who begins to nurse her child should start on the left side, as this is the source of all understanding.

Psychologist Lee Salk found 83 percent of right-handed and 78 percent of left-handed mothers held their babies on the left side.

Holding a baby on the left side frees up the baby's left ear to hear its mother's voice. Sounds that enter the left ear go to the right side of the brain, which processes tone, melody, and emotion.

‡ TEST YOUR PILLS

According to chemist Larry Royce, the vitamins, minerals, and other supplements you may be taking may be passing right through your body without doing you a bit of good! There's a simple test that can tell you whether or not your body has a chance of absorbing the pills you're taking.

Put the pill or capsule that you want to test in ½ cup of white vinegar. A small pill should disintegrate within a half hour, a big pill within an hour. If a pill is *enteric-coated* (check the label for those words), it may take more than an hour to disintegrate.

The vinegar represents your stomach acids. If it doesn't break down the pill, chances are your stomach acids won't either. If the pill *doesn't* break down, your body can't absorb it. If the pill *does* break down, it doesn't mean that your body *will* absorb it; it means that your body *can* (and, *hopefully*, will) absorb it.

‡ ARE YOU ABSORBING YOUR NUTRIENTS?

Ray C. Wunderlich, Jr., M.D., has a must-read essay on his Website (www.wunderlichcenter.com) called "The Real Doctor Asks the Most Important Question of ALL." It deals with the questions your doctor should be asking to best evaluate your state of health, and to help you practice preventive medicine.

And now for the most important question of all: Does your bowel movement mark the toilet bowl? Stools that adhere to the surface of the toilet bowl, leaving a mark, indicate faulty digestive capacity, usually of fat.

"No matter if one's diet is the best in the world, if not processed properly and absorbed," as Dr. Wunderlich poetically puts it, "one may feed the privy without being privy to nutrients that are being lost to that porcelain banquet."

‡ MICROWAVING SAVING VITAMINS

Fewer vitamins are destroyed when you prepare food in a microwave. Prevent food from burning by adding water—as little as possible to retain as many of the food's nutrients as possible. Also, cover foods while microwaving in order to reduce the zapping time and keep in more of the nutrients.

‡ LETTUCE: CHOOSE DARK GREEN

The darkest-green salad greens are the best. Romaine lettuce has two times as much folic acid, six times as much vitamin C, and eight times as much beta-carotene as iceberg lettuce. Spinach? Dark green. Watercress? Dark green. Collard greens, mustard greens: both dark green.

While you're at it, you may want to include parsley as a salad green, not just as a garnish. Parsley is rich in beta-carotene and vitamin C. It tastes good, too.

‡ WHEN TAKING ANTIBIOTICS . . .

Antibiotics have *no* discretion. They destroy the *good* as well as the *bad* bacteria. Replace the beneficial bacteria with *Lactobacillus acidophilus*. You can do that by eating yogurt—make sure the container says *Live* or *Active Culture with L. acidophilus*—or drinking acidophilus milk, or by taking an acidophilus supplement, available at health food stores. Whether you take a supplement, drink milk, or eat yogurt (fat-free is fine as long as it says it contains *L. acidophilus*), do it two hours *after* taking an antibiotic, making sure that it's also at least two hours *before* you have to take another dose of the antibiotic. Allow that amount of time before and after the antibiotic so that the acidophilus doesn't interfere with the work of the antibiotic.

Keep consuming acidophilus in some form for at least a

couple of weeks after you stop taking an antibiotic. It will help normalize the bacterial balance in the intestines, getting your digestive system working properly again.

‡ WHEY TO GO

You know that watery part that you spill out before taking a portion of yogurt? That's the whey and it has B vitamins and minerals, and little if any fat. Mix the whey into the yogurt so that it's part of your portion. (See the "Sensational Six" chapter for more yogurt information.)

‡ THE FULL MOON BOOM

Ralph Morris, professor of pharmacology at the University of Illinois Medical Center, did a study which led him to conclude that health problems may act up and can become more severe when there's a full moon.

‡ A FISHY STORY

Do you have any idea how the custom of serving a slice of lemon with fish first started? It wasn't to cut the fishy taste or to heighten the flavor. A long time ago, lemon was thought of more as a medicine than as a food. If someone swallowed a fish bone, the thinking was that the lemon juice was so strong that it would dissolve the bone.

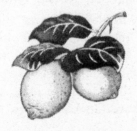

‡ MOLD ON FOOD

It's not a good thing. While it probably won't kill you, it can make you sick. If you see mold on any kind of food, do not give it the smell test to see if it has gone bad. Just a whiff of the mold spores can trigger an allergic or respiratory reaction. Get rid of soft foods or drinks that have even a hint of mold. If hard foods, like Swiss cheese, have mold, you can lop off the moldy part (play it safe and discard an inch all around the mold) and salvage the rest.

‡ FEVER: FRIEND OR FOE?

Thomas Sydenham, a seventeenth-century English physician, said, "Fever is Nature's engine which she brings into the field to remove her enemy."

It looks like research scientists are agreeing with Dr. Sydenham with regard to fevers below 104 degrees Fahrenheit.

Dr. Matthew J. Kluger at the Michigan Medical School and one of the leading researchers of fever therapy recommends that fever be allowed to run its course and that it may actually shorten the duration of an illness. Studies at the University of Texas Health Science Center in Dallas showed that fever supports antibiotic therapy. And researchers at Yale University School of Medicine proved that patients with fever are less contagious than those with the same infection but who have suppressed their fever with medication.

Dr. Ray C. Wunderlich, Jr., of the Wunderlich Center for Nutritional Medicine in St. Petersburg, Florida, says, "Mothers with hot babies in the middle of the night know that high fever paralyzes the household and may create extreme stress. Be sure the baby is not excessively clothed and blanketed. A twenty- to thirty-minute tepid bath may help the baby feel better and even feel like ingesting fluids or food."

‡ COMING TO YOUR SENSES

The average pair of eyes can distinguish nearly eight million differences in color.

The average pair of ears can discriminate among more than three hundred thousand tones.

The average nose can recognize ten thousand different odors.

There are thirteen hundred nerve endings per square inch in each average fingertip; the only parts of the body more sensitive to touch are the lips, the tongue, and the tip of the nose.

That covers four of our five senses. As for the fifth sense, well—everyone knows, there's no accounting for taste!

‡ THINK POSITIVE, LIVE LONGER

An optimistic approach may actually prolong your life, according to a study at the Mayo Clinic. Researchers studied patients for over thirty years and concluded that the pessimistic people run a 19 percent greater risk of death compared with the more optimistic ones. It's hard to put much credence in this study since so many variables come into play. The message here is that *optimistic* is a happier way to go through life than *pessimistic*, and it's much more pleasant for everyone around you.

‡ THE "REST" OF THE STORY

Everyone from your mother, mate, and doctor at one time or another probably suggested or insisted on "bed rest." A new study done by Michigan State University researchers and reported in the *Journal of Family Practice* says, "*Rest, not bed* rest." The difference between the two is important. When you rest, you slow down but keep moving. Bed rest implies staying still (in bed) for long periods of time. This can lead to muscle fatigue and even overall weakness. The researchers based their findings on close to six thousand patients with seventeen different medical conditions. Conclusion: It's good to get people out of bed as soon as possible. You may get out of bed, but you may still need rest. As your mother, mate, or doctor will tell you, "Don't overdo it!"

NOTE: Equal time is demanded by Dr. Ray C. Wunderlich, Jr., who reminds us that in some cases, "Don't under-do it!"

‡ DOCTOR'S FEE

In ancient China, doctors were paid when they kept their patients well. Believing it was their job to prevent illness, the doctors often paid patients who got sick.

Those were the good old days!

Recommended Reading

‡ **BODY POWER / BRAIN POWER**

Body for Life by Bill Phillips with Michael D'Orso (Harper-Collins, 1999). Twelve weeks to mental and physical strength. It promises a lot—*and* it delivers.

The Healing Power of the Mind by Rolf Alexander, M.D. (Healing Arts Press, 1989). Practical techniques for health and empowerment using imagination, desire, the power of suggestion, psychic influence, and more. Emphasizes our innate capacity for self-healing.

Your Miracle Brain by Jean Carper (HarperCollins, 2000). New scientific evidence reveals how you can use food and supplements to maximize your brain power, boost your memory, lift your mood, improve IQ and creativity, and prevent and reverse mental aging.

‡ **FOLK AND HOME REMEDIES**

Chicken Soup & Other Folk Remedies by Joan Wilen & Lydia Wilen (Ballantine Books, 2000). This handy reference book will help bring back memories of Grandma. It's filled with time-tested and doctor-approved remedies that turn your kitchen into a pharmacy.

Folk Remedies That Work by Joan Wilen & Lydia Wilen (HarperCollins, 1996). A useful, effective collection of safe, practical, doctor-approved New Age and age-old remedies.

‡ FOOD, HEALTHFUL EATING, AND WEIGHT PROGRAMS

Eating Well for Optimum Health—The Essential Guide to Food, Diet, and Nutrition by Andrew Weil, M.D. (Alfred A. Knopf, 2000). Worthwhile basic information and specific advice about making the right diet choices. Plus: eighty-five recipes!

Flax for Life! by Jade Beutler, R.R.T., R.C.P. (Apple Publishing, 1996). If the author's name seems familiar, it may be because of his contribution to the "flax oil" pages in our "Sensational Six Superfoods" chapter. Once you read about the benefits of flax oil, you may want this book, filled with 101 delicious recipes and tips.

Food Enzymes—The Missing Link to Radiant Health by Humbert Santillo, M.H., N.D. (Hohm Press, 1993). A practical and concise guide that explains why food enzymes from fruit and vegetable sources are essential for vitality and immunity. Weight control is also included.

40-30-30 Fat Burning Nutrition by Joyce and Gene Daoust (Wharton Publishing, 1996). The dietary hormonal connection to permanent weight loss and better health. Learn to balance nutrition that will help you burn fat while eating foods you enjoy.

GARLIC—Nature's Super Healer by Joan Wilen & Lydia Wilen (Prentice Hall, 1997). Discover the amazing power of garlic through remedies, recipes, and lore.

Healthy Nuts by Gene Spiller, Ph.D. (Avery Publishing Group, 2000). If you've read the "nuts" pages in our "Sensational Six Superfoods" chapter and it made you thirsty for more information, this book has it.

The Omega Diet by Artemis P. Simopoulos, M.D. and Jo Robinson (HarperCollins, 1999). A natural, time-tested eating plan that balances the fatty acids in your diet. Includes recipes and three weeks of meal plans to get you started.

SEAWEED—A Cook's Guide by Lesley Ellis (Fisher Books, 1998). Dare to try the tempting recipes using health-giving seaweed and sea vegetables.

7-Day Detox Miracle by Peter Bennett, N.D. and Stephen Barrie, N.D., with Sara Faye (Prima Publishing, 1999). Restore your mind and body's natural vitality with this life-enhancing program—and in only a week.

Understanding Fats & Oils by Michael T. Murray, N.D., and Jade Beutler, R.R., R.C.P. (Apple Publishing, 1996). This guide to healing with essential fatty acids has well-researched information, particularly about flax oil.

‡ HERBS

The Green Pharmacy by James A. Duke, Ph.D. (Rodale Press, 1997). A treasure filled with informative, enjoyable reading and herbal remedies for more than 120 conditions from the world's foremost authority on healing herbs.

The Herbal Home Spa by Greta Breedlove (Storey Books, 1998). Discover how to pamper your body from head to toe with refreshing wraps, rubs, lotions, masks, oils, and scrubs.

Herbal Remedy Gardens by Dorie Byers (Storey Books, 1999). A master gardener offers simple growing instructions for medicinal herbs, and tips for using them.

Natural Healing with Herbs by Humbart Santillo, N.D. (Hohm Press, 1984). Good reference book listing therapies for more than 140 common ailments and the properties of 120 commonly used herbs.

10 Essential Herbs by Lalitha Thomas (Hohm Press, 1996). Lalitha gets to the *root* of things. No one does it more thoroughly or better!

‡ JUST FOR MEN
The Viagra Alternative by Marc Bonnard, M.D. (Healing Arts Press, 1999). The complete guide to overcoming erectile dysfunction with natural, safe, and long-term cures. It also contains an analysis of Viagra and its competitors.

‡ JUST FOR WOMEN
The Estrogen Alternative by Raquel Martin with Judi Gerstung, D.C. (Healing Arts Press, 1997). If you are concerned about PMS, endometriosis, osteoporosis, or menopause, this book offers information on natural hormone therapy with botanical progesterone. You may want to discuss it with your gynecologist.

Your Pregnancy—Every Woman's Guide by Glade B. Curtis, M.D., OB/GYN (Fisher Books, 1999). Helpful tips, facts, and answers to questions you may have during your pregnancy.

‡ NEW AGE AND AGE-OLD (MOSTLY ALTERNATIVE) THERAPIES
Alternative Medicine: The Definitive Guide, compiled by The Burton Goldberg Group (Future Medicine Publishing, 1994). This huge book is brimming with information from

almost four hundred leading alternative health professionals who share their effective therapies.

Ayurvedic Secrets to Longevity and Total Health by Peter Anselmo with James S. Brooks, M.D. (Prentice Hall, 1996). A how-to guide to the ancient healing art of Ayurvedic medicine.

Common Scents by Lorrie Hargis (Woodland Publishing, 1999). A practical guide to aromatherapy; using essential oils to improve health.

Creative Healing by Michael Samuels, M.D., and Mary Rockwood Lane, R.N. (HarperCollins, 1998). Through guided imagery, personal stories, and practical exercises, learn to find your "inner artist healer" and improve your health, attitude, and sense of well-being.

The Healing Power of Color by Betty Wood (Destiny Books, 1998). Using color to improve your mental, physical, and spiritual well-being.

Healing Visualizations by Gerald Epstein, M.D. (Bantam Books, 1989). Dr. Epstein, a psychiatrist and pioneer in waking dream therapy, helps you create health through imagery in easy-to-do, carefully explained visualizations.

Laffirmations—1,001 Ways to Add Humor to Your Life and Work by Joel Goodman (Health Communications, Inc., 1995). Daily thought-provoking quotations, questions, and tips to bring more laughter into your life.

The Power of Touch by Phyllis K. Davis, Ph.D. (Hay House, Inc., 1999). Learn how even the simplest forms of touch influence your behavior and enrich the lives of everyone in your life. There are also lots of helpful activities and useful ideas.

Prayer, Faith and Healing—Cure Your Body, Heal Your Mind and Restore Your Soul by Kenneth Winston Caine and Brian Paul Kaufman (Rodale Press, 1999). Over five hundred ways to use the power of belief, from America's leading pastors, counselors, doctors, and health researchers.

Qigong—Essence of the Healing Dance by Garri Garripoli and Friends (Health Communications, Inc., 1999). Qigong (pronounced *chee gung*) is an ancient Chinese health care modality. You can learn how your own bioelectric force can be used for self-healing or healing others.

The Ultimate Healing System by Donald Lepore, N.D. (Woodland Publishing, 1985). An illustrated guide to muscle testing (bio-kinesiology) and a variety of therapies to help correct problematic conditions.

Your Own Perfect Medicine by Martha M. Christy (Future Medicine Publishing, Inc., 1994). A comprehensive look at the mainstream medical uses of urine therapy, proving its ability to help cure many illnesses.

‡ PETS

Natural Pet Cures by Dr. John Heinerman (Prentice Hall, 1998). The author, one of the world's leading authorities on natural healing for people, now shares all-natural remedies for sixty-three common health problems that affect dogs and cats.

‡ SPECIFIC HEALTH CHALLENGES

An Alternative Medicine Definitive Guide to Cancer by W. John Diamond, M.D., and W. Lee Cowden, M.D., with Burton Goldberg (Future Medicine Publishing, Inc., 1997). Cancer can be reversed. This important, lifesaving book tells how, using clinically proven complementary and alternative therapies. Thirty-seven physicians explain their proven, safe, nontoxic, and successful treatments for reversing cancer.

Asthma Free in 21 Days by Kathryn Shafer, Ph.D., and Fran Greenfield, M.A. (HarperCollins, 2000). This breakthrough mind-body healing program is an absolute must for any adult or child with asthma.

Beyond Aspirin by Thomas Newmark and Paul Schulick (Hohm Press, 2000). The COX-2 medical revolution! Nature's answer to arthritis, cancer, and Alzheimer's disease.

Enhancing Fertility Naturally by Nicky Wesson (Healing Arts Press, 1999). Holistic therapies for a successful pregnancy.

Naturally Healthy Skin by Stephanie Tourles (Storey Books, 1999). A complete program of easy-to-follow treatments, including tips and techniques, for clear skin.

The Pain Cure by Dharma Singh Khalsa, M.D., with Cameron Stauth (Warner Books, 1999). The proven medical program— uniting conventional and alternative therapies—to help end chronic pain due to migraines, carpal tunnel, back, and more.

The Prozac Alternative by Ran Knishinsky (Healing Arts Press, 1998). An important source of natural remedies— St.-John's-wort, kava, gingko, 5-HTP, homepathic medicine— to treat anxiety, stress, and depression.

7 Weeks to Emotional Healing by Joan Mathews Larson, Ph.D. (Ballantine Books, 1999). Proven natural formulas for eliminating depression, anxiety, fatigue, and anger from your life.

‡ VITAMINS AND OTHER SUPPLEMENTS

Dr. Heinerman's Encyclopedia of Nature's Vitamins and Minerals by John Heinerman, Ph.D. (Prentice Hall, 1998). Learn the properties of many vitamins and minerals, the best food sources for them, and preparation tips.

The Natural Pharmacist: Natural Health Bible, edited by Steven Bratman, M.D., and David Kroll, Ph.D. (Prima Publishing, 1999). Comprehensive A–Z guide of herbs, vitamins, and other supplements, and their uses for more than two hundred health conditions.

Sources

‡ HERBAL PRODUCTS AND MORE

Atlantic Spice Company
2 Shore Road
P.O. Box 205
North Truro, MA 02652
Note: Wholesale to
the public.

Free Catalog
Tel: 800 / 316-7965
Fax: 508 / 487-2550
Website: www.atlantic
spice.com

Blessed Herbs
109 Barre Plains Road
Oakham, MA 01068

Free Catalog
Tel: 800 / 489-4372
Fax: 508 / 882-3755
Email:blessedherbs@
blessedherbs.com

Dial Herbs
P.O. Box 39
Fairview, UT 84629

Free Catalog
Tel: 800 / 288-4618
435 / 427-9476
Fax: 435 / 427-9448
Website: www.dialdist.com

Flower Power Herbs
and Roots, Inc.
406 East 9th Street
New York, NY 10009

Tel: 212 / 982-6664
Website: www.flower
power.net

Great American Natural Products
4121 16th Street North
St. Petersburg, FL 33703

Free Catalog
Tel: 800 / 323-4372
Fax: 727 / 522-6457

Haussmann's Herbs & Naturals
220 Market Street
Philadelphia, PA 19106

Free Catalog
Tel: 800 / 235-5522
      215 / 627-1168
Fax: 215 / 629-0339

Indiana Botanic Gardens
3401 West 37th Avenue
Hobart, IN 46325

Free Catalog
Tel: 800 / 644-8327
      219 / 947-4040
Fax: 219 / 947-4148
Website: www.botanic
      health.com

Mountain Top Herbs, Inc.
P.O. Box 970004
Orem, UT 84097-0004

Tel: 877 / KIT-TALK
         (548-8255)
Website: www.herb
      kit.com

Nature's Apothecary
P.O. Box 17976
Boulder, CO 80308

Free Catalog
Tel: 800 / 999-7422
      303 / 664-1600
Fax: 303 / 664-5106
Website: www.natures
      apothecary.com

New Chapter, Inc.
P.O. Box 1947
22 High Street
Brattleboro, VT 05301

Free Catalog
Tel: 800 / 543-7279
      802 / 257-0018
Fax: 802 / 257-0018
Website: www.new
      chapter.com

Old Amish Herbal Remedies
4141 Irish Street North
St. Petersburg, FL 33703

Free Catalog
Tel: 813 / 521-4372
Fax: 727 / 522-6457

Penn Herb Co. Ltd.
10601 Decatur Road-Suite 2
Philadelphia, PA 19154

Free Catalog
Tel: 800 / 523-9971
Fax: 215 / 632-7945
Website: www.penn
herb.com

San Francisco Herb Company
250 14th Street
San Francisco, CA 94103
Note: Wholesale to the public.

Free Catalog
Tel: 800 / 227-4530
Fax: 415 / 861-4440
Website: www.sfherb.com

‡ GEMS AND NEW AGE PRODUCTS AND GIFTS

Beyond the Rainbow
P.O. Box 110
Ruby, NY 12475

Tel: 914 / 336-4609
Fax: 914 / 336-0953
Website: www.rainbow
crystal.com

Crystal Way
2335 Market Street
San Francisco, CA 94114

Tel: 800 / 453-HEAL (4325)
    415 / 861-6511
Fax: 415 / 861-4229
Website: www.crystalway.com

Divine Intervention
1580 Main Street #270
Hesperia, CA 92345

Tel: 800 / 863-3442
Fax: 760 / 947-4093
Website: www.divine
intervention.com

Pacific Spirit
1334 Pacific Avenue
Forest Grove, OR 97116

Free Catalog
Tel: 800 / 634-9057
Fax: 503 / 357-1669
Website: www.mystictrader.com

‡ VITAMINS, NUTRITIONAL SUPPLEMENTS, AND MORE

Freeda Vitamins
36 East 41st Street
New York, NY 10017
Note: All products are
100 percent kosher, yeast-free, vegetarian, and
Feingold-approved for
hyperactive children.

Free Catalog
Tel: 800 / 777-3737
     212 / 685-4980
Fax: 212 / 685-7297
Website: www.freeda
    vitamins.com

Nature's Distributors, Inc.
16508 E. Laser Drive,
Building B
Fountain Hills,
    AZ 85268-6512

Free Catalog
Tel: 800 / 624-7114
Fax: 480 / 837-8420
Website: www.natures
    distributors.com

NutriCology Inc.
30806 Santana Street
Hayward, CA 94544

Free Catalog
Tel: 800 / 545-9960
Fax: 510 / 487-8682
Website: www.nutricology.com

Nutrition Coalition, Inc.
P.O. Box 3001
Fargo, ND 58108

Free Information on
    Willard Water
Tel: 800 / 447-4793
Fax: 218 / 236-6753
Website: www.willardswater.com

Puritan's Pride
1233 Montauk Highway
P.O. Box 9001
Oakdale, NY 11769–9001

Free Catalog
Tel: 800 / 645-1030
Fax: 631 / 471-5693
Website: www.puritan.com

Superior Nutritionals Inc.
1150 94th Avenue North
St. Petersburg, FL 33702

Tel: 800 / 717-RUNN (7866)
    727 / 577-4344
Fax: 727 / 577-3166

Specializes in well-researched,
  high-quality, physician-tested products.

TriMedica International, Inc.   Free Catalog
1895 So. Los Feliz Drive   Tel: 800 / 800-8849
Tempe, AZ 85282   Fax: 480 / 346-3191
                                  Website: www.trimedica.com

Vitamins.com   Free Catalog
2924 Telestar Court   Tel: 800 / 741-8273
Falls Church, VA 22042   Website: www.vitamins.com

Vitamin Shoppe.com   Free Catalog
4700 Westside Avenue   Tel: 888 / 880-3055
North Bergen, NJ 07047   Fax: 800 / 476-3851
                                  Website:
                                    www.vitaminshoppe.com

‡ NATURAL FOODS AND MORE

Barlean's Organic Oils   Free Catalog &
4936 Lake Terrell Road   Flax Oil Information
Ferndale, WA 98248   Tel: 800 / 445-FLAX (3529)
                                  Fax: 800 / 551-9879
                                  Website: www.barleans.com

Crusoe Island Natural Foods   Free Catalog
267 Rt. 89 South   Tel: 800 / 724-2233
Savannah, NY 13146-9711   315 / 365-3949
                                  Fax: 315 / 365-2690
                                  Website:
                                    www.crusoeisland.com

Gold Mine Natural Food Co.   Free Catalog
7805 Arjons Drive   Tel: 800 / 475-FOOD (3663)
San Diego, CA 92126   Fax: 619 / 695-0811

Website: www.
goldminenaturalfood.com

Jaffe Bros. Natural Foods, Inc.
28560 Lilac Road
Valley Center, CA
92082-0636

Free Catalog
Tel: 760 / 749-1133
Fax: 760 / 749-1282
Website: www.organicfruits
andnuts.com

‡ BEE PRODUCTS AND MORE

C.C. Pollen
3627 E. Indian School
Road / Suite 209
Phoenix, AZ 85018

Free Literature & Product List
Tel: 800 / 875-0096
602 / 957-0096
Fax: 602 / 381-3130
Website: www.ccpollen.com

Health from the Hive
Bee Supplies & Products
James Hagemeyer
("Mr. Bee Pollen")
5337 Highway 411
Madisonville, TN 37354

Tel: 423 / 442-2038
Website: www.bee-pollen.com

Montana Naturals
19994 Highway 93
Arlee, MT 59821

Tel: 800 / 872-7218
Fax: 800 / 239-4819

‡ PET FOOD AND PRODUCTS

All The Best Pet Care
8050 Lake City Way
Seattle, WA 98115

Free Catalog
Tel: 800 / 962-8266
206 / 522-1667
Fax: 206 / 522-1132
Website:
www.allthebestpetcare.com

Golden Tails
6509 Transit Road, Suite B2
Bowmansville, NY 14026

Tel: 716 / 681-6986
Fax: 716 / 681-6958
Website: www.goldentails.com

Halo Purely For Pets
3438 E. Lake Road, #14
Palm Harbor, FL 34685

Free Catalog & Animal
Care Booklet
Tel: 800 / 426-4256
Fax: 813 / 891-6328
Website: www.halopets.com

Harbingers of a New Age
717 E. Missoula Avenue
Troy, MT 59935–9609

Free Catalog
Tel: 406 / 295-4944
Fax: 406 / 295-7603
Website: www.
montanasat.net/vegepet

‡ HEALTH-RELATED PRODUCTS

Inner Balance—Natural
Solutions For Health
360 Interlocken Blvd.,
   Suite 300
Broomfield, CO 80021

Free Catalog
Tel: 800 / 482-3608
Fax: 800 / 456-1139
Website: www.gaiam.com

InteliHealth Healthy Home
97 Commerce Way
Dover, DE 19904

Free Catalog
Tel: 800 / 988-1127
Fax: 800 / 676-3299
Website: www.intelihealth.com

Perfect Balance For Mind,
Body and Soul
7101 Winnetka Avenue North
P.O. Box 9437
Minneapolis, MN 55440-9437

Free Catalog
Tel: 800 / 729-9000

Website: www.damark.com

Self Care Catalog
104 Challenger Drive
Portland, TN 37148

Free Catalog
Tel: 800 / 345-3371
Fax: 800 / 345-4021
Website: www.selfcare.com

‡ HEALTH-RELATED TRAVEL PRODUCTS AND MORE

Magellan's
  (Essentials for the Traveler)
110 West Sola Street
Santa Barbara, CA 93101

Free Catalog
Tel: 800 / 962-4943
Fax: 805 / 962-4940
Website: www.magellans.com

‡ MACROBIOTIC FOODS AND SPECIALTY COOKWARE

Mountain Ark
  Trading Company
799 Old Leicester Highway
Asheville, NC 28806

Free Catalog
Tel: 800 / 438-4730
Fax: 828 / 252-9479
Website:
  www.mountainark.com

‡ WHOLESALE/RETAIL HEALTH APPLIANCES

Acme Equipment
1024 Concert Avenue
Spring Hill, FL 34609

Free Catalog
Tel: 800 / 201-0706
Fax: 352 / 683-7740

‡ AROMATHERAPY, FLOWER ESSENCES, AND MORE

Aromaland
1326 Rufina Circle
Santa Fe, NM 87505

Free Catalog
Tel: 800 / 933-5267
Fax: 505 / 438-7223
Website: www.aromaland.com

Aroma Vera
5901 Rodeo Road
Los Angeles, CA 90016

Free Catalog
Tel: 800 / 669-9514
    310 / 204-3392
Fax: 310 / 204-2746
Website: www.aromavera.com

Flower Essence Services
P.O. Box 1769
Nevada City, CA 95959

Free Catalog
Tel: 800 / 548-0075
    530 / 265-0258
Fax: 530 / 265-6467
Website:
    www.floweressence.com

‡ SERVICES

Ailment Information Including Holistic Alternatives

LaVerne and Steve Ross are co-founders of the World Research Foundation. They have an incredible service. For a nominal fee, they will do a search (which includes five thousand international medical journals) and provide you with the newest holistic and conventional treatments and diagnostic techniques on most any condition. The Foundation's library of more than ten thousand books, periodicals, and research reports is available to the public free of charge. Write, call, fax, or visit their Website.

World Research Foundation
41 Bell Rock Plaza
Sedona, AZ 86351

Tel: 520 / 284-3300
Fax: 520 / 284-3530
Website: www.wrf.org

Product Safety

The U.S. Consumer Product Safety Commission has an around-the-clock hotline with information on harmful products. With paper and pen in hand, call: 800 / 638-2772; Maryland residents, call: 800 / 492-8104.

Check up on Specialists

The American Board of Medical Specialties has a toll-free number for you to call when you want to make sure that a "specialist" is just that. When you call, give them the doctor's name, and they will tell you whether the doctor is listed in a specialty and the year of certification. Call weekdays, between 9 A.M. – 6 P.M. EST: 800 / 776-CERT (2378).

Take Advantage of Your Tax Dollars

The Consumer Information Catalog lists more than two hundred free and low-cost publications from Uncle Sam—on everything from saving money, staying healthy, and getting federal benefits to buying a home and handling consumer complaints.

There are three easy ways to get your free copy of the catalog:

- Call toll-free: 888 / 8-PUEBLO (878-3256), weekdays 9 A.M. to 8 P.M. EST.
- Send your name and address to Consumer Information Catalog, Pueblo, CO 81009.
- Go online to check out and order the catalog through the Consumer Information Center's Website at www.pueblo.gsa.gov. While you're there, you can read, print out, or download any CIC publication for free.

Health-Related Websites

Before we start www-ing down the page, there's something you should know, and probably already do: You can't always trust the information you get on the Internet. Since we're talking about "your health," it can be mighty dangerous to accept and use wrong advice. Our advice is to take whatever information you get online that seems appropriate for your condition, and show it to and/or discuss it with your health professional.

There's something else you may already know, but if not, you should. There's an organization called the HON (Health On the Net) Foundation (**www.hon.ch**), associated with the University Hospitals of Geneva. HON is like the Better Business Bureau for medical Websites. Their prestigious governing body certifies sites that abide by eight user-protecting principles. So, if HON gives a site its stamp of approval, you will see it on the site, and while you may be able to trust the integrity of the information a bit more, still be sure to check out any and all advice with your health professional.

HON is not the only organization certifying Websites. There's the Internet Healthcare Coalition (**www.ihc.net**) and Health Internet Ethics (Hi-Ethics), founded in part by former surgeon general C. Everett Koop (**www.healthwise. org/Hi-EthicsHome.htm**).

At these three Websites, you'll find direct links to established (and certified, of course) health sites—many of the ones listed below.

www.americanheart.org
American Heart Association National Center
Education and information on fighting heart disease and stroke.

www.arfa.org
The American Running Association
News, tips, articles, membership information, fitness links, and free sample *Running & FitNews* newsletter.

www.askdrweil.com (or) **www.drweil.com**
Dr. Andrew Weil answers health questions asked by emailers. User-friendly archives.

www.cancer.org
American Cancer Society
Education and information.

www.certifieddoctor.org
Online version of American Board of Medical Specialties
Public Education Program's physician locator and information service.

www.chid.nih.gov
Combined Health Information Database for National Institutes of Health, Centers for Disease Control and Prevention, and Health Resources and Services Administration.

www.clinicaltrials.gov
A service of the National Institutes of Health
Current information about clinical research studies, linking patients to medical research.

www.eFit.com
Health and fitness site with lots going on. Free personalized weight management, nutrition, and exercise program. Type in your zip code and find the closest gyms and healthy-menu restaurants.

www.familydoctor.co.nz
Health information by practicing doctors.

www.fda.gov
Food and Drug Administration.

www.healthfinder.gov
U.S. Department of Health and Human Services
The site is linked to other agencies and self-help and support groups.

www.healthweb.org
Provides links to specific, evaluated information resources selected by librarians and professionals at leading academic medical centers in the Midwest.

www.healthyideas.com
Prevention's Website has herbal remedies, vitamin databases, alternative medicine news, advice from naturopathic doctors, and lots more.

www.kidshealth.org
Created by pediatric medical experts at the Nemours Foundation.

www.mealsforyou.com
Thousands of recipes, meal plans, complete nutritional information. Look up recipes by name, ingredient, or nutritional content. Recipes adjust for number of servings; shopping list itemizes ingredients.

www.merck.com
Searchable online version of the Merck Manual of Medical Information.

www.medlineplus.gov
National Library of Medicine's Medline Plus
Health information selected by the National Library of Medicine from a database of more than four thousand medical journals.

www.oncolink.upenn.edu
The University of Pennsylvania's cancer information site with related information links.

www.siu.edu/departments/bushea
Your Health Is Your Business
Links to many health sites.

www.soyfoods.com
Monthly newsletter, soy research information, U.S. soyfoods directory, recipe books, food manufacturing information.

www.talksoy.com
Soy recipes and health and nutrition information.

www.wellweb.com
WellnessWeb
A comprehensive health and medical information clearinghouse, including conventional and alternative medicine, nutrition, and fitness, and late-breaking medical research on nutrition and fitness.

www.wunderlichcenter.com
Dr. Ray C. Wunderlich, Jr., known as "The Real Doctor" in honor of his pioneering contributions in the alternative medicine movement, is dedicated to promoting nutritional and preventive medicine at the Wunderlich Center for Nutritional Medicine in St. Petersburg, Florida. The Website has his informative and humorous health articles.

Index